A Celebration of General Practice

Edited by

Mayur Lakhani MRCP FRCGP

Chair of Communications and Publishing Network
Royal College of General Practitioners

Foreword by
Professor Dame Lesley Southgate

Radcliffe Medical Press

Radcliffe Medical Press Ltd
18 Marcham Road
Abingdon
Oxon OX14 1AA
United Kingdom

www.radcliffe-oxford.com
The Radcliffe Medical Press electronic catalogue and online ordering facility. Direct
sales to anywhere in the world.

British Library Cataloguing in Publication Data

A catalogue record for this book is available from the British Library.

ISBN 1 85775 923 0

Typeset by Advance Typesetting Ltd, Oxfordshire
Printed and bound by TJ International Ltd, Padstow, Cornwall

Contents

List of contributors

Maureen Baker DM, FRCGP
Honorary Secretary of Council, Royal College of General Practitioners

Richard Baker OBE, MD, FRCGP
Professor of Quality in Health Care and Director, Clinical Governance Research and Development Unit, Department of General Practice & Primary Health Care, University of Leicester, Leicester, UK

Yvonne H Carter OBE, MD, FRCGP, FMedSci
Professor of General Practice and Primary Care, St Bartholomew's and the Queen Mary's School of Medicine and Dentistry, London, UK

Steve Field MMEd, ILTM, FRCGP, DRCOG
Honorary Professor of Medical Education, University of Warwick; Chairman of Education Network, Royal College of General Practitioners and Regional Postgraduate Dean, West Midlands, UK

Per Fugelli MD, FRCGP
Professor of Social Medicine, Institute of General Practice and Community Medicine, University of Oslo, Norway

David Haslam FRCGP
Chairman of Council, Royal College of General Practitioners

Amanda Howe MD, FRCGP
Professor of Primary Care, School of Medicine, Health Policy and Practice, University of East Anglia and Chair of Research, Royal College of General Practitioners

Sally Hull MSc, MRCP, FRCGP
Senior Clinical Lecturer, Department of General Practice and Primary Care, Queen Mary's School of Medicine and Dentistry, London, UK

Claire Jackson MA
College Archivist, Royal College of General Practitioners

Mayur Lakhani MRCP, FRCGP
Chair of Communications and Publishing Network, Royal College of General Practitioners

Ian R McWhinney OC, MD, FRCP, FRCGP, FCFP
Professor Emeritus of Family Medicine, University of Western Ontario, Canada

Joe Neary MSc, FRCGP
Chair of Clinical and Special Projects Network, Royal College of General Practitioners

Professor Sir Denis Pereira Gray OBE, DSc, FRCP, FRCGP, FMedSci
President, Royal College of General Practitioners, 1997–2000; Chairman, Academy of Medical Royal Colleges, 2000–2002

Mike Pringle CBE, MD, FRCP, FRCGP, FMedSci
Former Chairman of Council, Royal College of General Practitioners and Head of School of Community Health Sciences, University of Nottingham, Nottingham, UK

Barbara Starfield MD, MPH, FRCGP
University Distinguished Professor, The Johns Hopkins University School of Medicine and Bloomberg School of Public Health, Baltimore, Maryland, USA

Chris van Weel MD, PhD, FRCGP
Professor of General Practice and Head of Department of General Practice, University Medical Centre, Nijmegen, the Netherlands

Patricia Wilkie PhD
Lay representative, Academy of Medical Royal Colleges and formerly Chair of the Patient Liaison Group, Royal College of General Practitioners

Foreword from the President of the Royal College of General Practitioners

A Celebration of General Practice is an exciting collection of essays on general practice at the beginning of the new century. At a time of continuing debates on the nature and effectiveness of healthcare provision, a group of distinguished authors present their views on the value and distinctive contribution of general practice. This is not just a snapshot in time. In tackling their particular theme, each author seeks not only to place their work in a historical and contemporary context, but looks to the future with confidence and a firm belief in the enduring value of the discipline. The essays are a pleasing mixture of scholarship and creative writing.

The emphasis throughout is on achievement and success. Denis Pereira Gray concentrates on the achievements of the College, Mike Pringle on the value of general practice to the NHS, whilst Richard Baker takes as his theme quality and standards. Steve Field looks at the education and training of general practitioners and Amanda Howe and Yvonne Carter examine the role of the general practitioner as a teacher. There are essays on the research basis of general practice from Yvonne Carter and Amanda Howe, on information management from Joe Neary, on women in general practice from Maureen Baker and on the doctor–patient relationship from Sally Hull. Patricia Wilkie broadens out the theme of the doctor–patient relationship in her essay on the value of general practice to the public. Ian McWhinney in 'The essence of general practice', Per Fugelli in 'The general practitioner and the spirits of time' and Claire Jackson and Mayur Lakhani in 'General practice: evolution or revolution' have written essays on the broader theme of the history and philosophy of general practice. David Haslam writes on the future GP. Barbara Starfield and Chris van Weel write from the perspective of international primary care, in their respective contributions on the effectiveness of primary healthcare and international perspectives.

For the freshness and imaginativeness of the authors' approach, for the depth of scholarship, for the variety of the contributions and above all for the firm conviction that each author holds that general practice fulfils a unique and unparalleled role in primary healthcare provision in this country, I cannot recommend this book highly enough to you. It will stimulate, enthuse and delight you.

Professor Dame Lesley Southgate DBE MClinSci FRCP FMedSci PRCGP
RCGP, London
June 2003

Preface

On 19 November 1952, a College of General Practitioners (later the Royal College of General Practitioners, RCGP) was founded in London and became the first academic body for general practitioners (GPs) in Europe: 2002 therefore marked the golden jubilee of the RCGP. I had the privilege of chairing the College's 50th anniversary committee from 2001 to 2002. During September 2002 we ran the first ever public awareness campaign[1] about general practice. The College had wanted to explain the strengths of family medicine and celebrate the achievements of GPs.

This book is an extension of that theme, the main audience being the wider health community. It is intended to mark the development and achievements of general practice-based primary healthcare in the United Kingdom (UK). This publication is therefore a collection of essays that looks at distinguished and distinguishing aspects of general practice. It is often not appreciated how much progress has been made in general practice – a word that is frequently used is 'transformation'. This becomes obvious when one examines the difference now and 50 years ago in how primary healthcare is organised, the quality and standards and range of services provided, the premises from which GPs practice, the use of information management and technology where general practice leads the way in the National Health Service (NHS), and the development of research and teaching.

This book is not a history of the RCGP – excellent publications on this already exist.[2] It may be hard to understand the need to 'celebrate' general practice – indeed this may be regarded as defensive. However, few people realise the struggle faced in establishing the RCGP and getting general practice *accepted* and respected as a discipline.

The strategic aim of the book – which guided the selection of material – can therefore be summarised as follows:

- to celebrate the establishment of the discipline of general practice
- to consider the influence and leadership of GPs and general practice in the wider health community
- to mark the contribution of the RCGP to developments in general practice and primary healthcare
- to note aspects of general practice that are notable for their wider applications and influence, e.g. use of computers for medical records and the study of communication and consultation skills
- to improve the understanding of general practice.

The book is intended to demonstrate the value of general practice to the public and the health service. Whilst the book has much of its material from the UK, we have included international issues, thinking and authors. This is of necessity a selected view of the development of the discipline of general practice, but we feel that is important to examine some of the reasons which led to the creation of the College and to explore how this might assist us in coping with the considerable challenges faced by general practice now. There was much more material that we could have included – I am sure that pundits will argue over the choice of material and the focus for the chapters. I cannot pretend that the coverage is comprehensive – indeed it is not intended to be. What I hope the book has done is capture the key areas of the practice of medicine where general practice has particular cause to celebrate. There is a degree of overlap between the chapters in the book which is intentional as each chapter can be read on its own.

Here is something about each chapter to explain why we chose a particular theme. I asked Professor Emeritus Ian McWhinney to write about 'The essence of general practice'. I felt this was necessary to explain what was special and different about our discipline. That general practice works and contributes to effective and efficient healthcare is shown convincingly by Professor Barbara Starfield in her chapter entitled 'The effectiveness of primary healthcare'. Professor Richard Baker shares with us progress made in raising standards of patient care in a chapter on the evolution of quality in primary healthcare and the current state of play. In 'Celebrating European cooperation in general practice', Professor Chris van Weel highlights the importance of learning and sharing in the European – and wider – family medicine communities. A further chapter extols the value of general practice to the NHS, by Professor Mike Pringle. I asked Patricia Wilkie to write about the special place of general practice and GPs in society. Her contribution as a lay member delineates the value of general practice to the public.

A special cause for celebration is the study of the doctor–patient consultation which is at the heart of general practice, so I have commissioned a chapter on this by Dr Sally Hull. Dr Hull writes about the study of the doctor–patient relationship, emphasising communication skills and patient-centred care, and its influence in primary care and effect on the whole of medical practice.

In 'Fifty years of research in general practice', Professors Yvonne Carter and Amanda Howe describe the great strides made in establishing general practice as an academic discipline underpinned by a research foundation. Some 3900 practices (one-third of all practices) are involved in community-based under-graduate education in the UK! I felt that this contribution must be recognised and explored further. Amanda Howe and Yvonne Carter do this in their chapter 'The general practitioner as a teacher'. Professor Steve Field writes about the story of general practice postgraduate training and education, detailing the development of vocational training and considering its future and links with continuing professional developments. Professor Sir Denis Pereira Gray writes about 'The creation and achievements of the RCGP'.

Dr Maureen Baker, in her chapter 'Careers: the contribution of women to general practice', highlights the substantial role played by women in general practice, both in service delivery and in leadership roles in the health community. Dr Joe Neary, in 'Achievements in record keeping: the use of information management and technology', looks at the development of record keeping in general practice from Lloyd George records to modern computer systems, stressing how general practice has led the way.

And so to the future! In 'The future of general practice', David Haslam gives us a glimpse of what the future GP role might be, to reflect the developing vision of the RCGP and considering issues such as skill mix, access, personal care and continuity. Per Fugelli, in 'The general practitioner and the spirits of time', tells us that the 'the body of GPs must communicate with society, be interactive with the modern health soul'. Finally, in my chapter written together with Claire Jackson, 'General practice: evolution or revolution?', we attempt to pull together all the various themes and invite readers to think about revitalisation and renaissance of general practice.

This book is intended to 'speak up' for general practice. I hope that the material in this book has done justice to this. I hope it will enable GPs and organisations of family medicine to remain 'true to the essence of general practice' and to continue to argue for this cause. Per Fugelli states that 'the GP is the streetwise guy of medicine' and that 'no one is more able to survive in the evolution of medicine than general practitioners'.

Mayur Lakhani FRCGP
RCGP, London
June 2003

References

1   National General Practice Week. http://www.rcgp.org.uk

2   Pereira Gray DJ (1992) *Forty Years On: the story of the first forty years of the Royal College of General Practitioners*. Atalink, London.

Acknowledgements

I am very grateful to all the authors for working to tight deadlines and for being so generous with their time and commitment to this book. I am grateful to Dr Peter Toon, former editor of RCGP publications, who undertook the initial development of this publication that marks the achievements of general practice. Helen Farrelly, Simone Jemmott, Jane Austin, Tamzyn Wigglesworth and Kylie Richards from the Communications and Publishing Network at the RCGP gave me invaluable support and advice. Lesley Fogg, my personal assistant, for her work on this book at the all-important initial commissioning stage. The publishers, Radcliffe Medical Press, have also been very helpful in supporting this project. My colleagues on the 50th Anniversary and Heritage Committee (chaired by Dr Lotte Newman) for their many useful comments and suggestions – their encouragement was invaluable. Dr Bill Reith, Chairman of the Scottish Council, for permission to use the Per Fugelli peripatetic lecture, 'The general practitioner and the spirits of time', given in Scotland. I would like to thank in particular my wife and children.

A collection of essays to mark the
50th Anniversary of the
Royal College of General Practitioners

CHAPTER 1

The essence of general practice

Ian R McWhinney

The essence of general practice is an unconditional and open-ended commitment to one's patients. We define ourselves in terms of this relationship. Clinicians in other fields form relationships with patients, but their commitment is to patients who have a disease or problem within their speciality. Most other fields define themselves in terms of content: diseases, organ systems or technologies. In general practice, the relationship is usually prior to content. We commit ourselves to patients before we know what their illnesses will be. It is, of course, possible to arrive at a content of general practice, based on common conditions presenting to GPs at a particular time and place, but the content for a particular doctor is the conditions their patients happen to have.

Karl Popper[1] said that scientific disciplines are defined by the problems they address, not by their subject matter. In applied disciplines like clinical medicine, this means that a field must first define its place in the scheme of things. In all clinical disciplines, subject matter changes with time. Morbidity patterns change; technologies become obsolete and are replaced by others; a discipline may became redundant if its problems are solved or taken over by other disciplines. General practice is no exception, and must show what remains constant as the content changes.

The commitment of a GP is to a person, not to 'a person with a certain disease'. If we are to fill our place, it is crucial that our commitment be unconditional. Patients should feel confident that they will never be told 'this is not my field'. We must not say: I will be your doctor as long as you don't have acquired immunodeficiency syndrome (AIDS), or as long as you are not house-bound, or dying, or too complicated. If we allow this to happen, general practice could break into a hundred fragments. The unconditional nature of the com-mitment means that the relationship is open-ended: it is ended only by death, by geographical separation, by mutual consent or, in some cases, by withdrawal of one of the parties.

A number of things flow from this relationship. If successful, it allows intimacy and friendship to grow, based on a mutual interest in the patient's health and well-being. This is not the same as a social friendship, though a social friend or acquaintance may also be a patient. At its best, the relationship will be one of trust; though trust has to be earned and is fragile as well as precious. The relationship deepens our knowledge of our patients' lives,[2] though we must always be prepared for surprises. We may not know our patients as well as we think we do. Cumulative knowledge in a long-term relationship gives us great advantages. It means that every new event can be understood in the context of a life story. The readiness to listen and respond to any problem a patient may present forms the basis of one of the GP's key skills: the assessment of undifferentiated clinical problems. Forming relationships when patients are healthy positions us for preventive practices across a spectrum, from health education to early diagnosis.[3]

Of course, things do not always go so smoothly. Relationships often end when patients or doctors move away. Relationships break down and may be better ended. Trust may fail: we all fail patients at times. Sometimes we are forgiven, sometimes not. Some patients do not want a relationship, let alone an intimate one. Others come to value the relationship only when they feel the need of one. Some relationships become distant when patients gravitate to secondary care with cancer or AIDS or mental illness, or to walk-in clinics or alternative medicine. Because of our own limitations there are times when we have to transfer care to a specialist, sometimes for a long period, but if the patient needs us again, we can still be there for them. The relationship is not ended.

The relationship between practitioner and patient is like others in which there are strong moral obligations and mutual commitments, such as those between parent and child and teacher and student. Although continuity is important in all of them, it is not simply a matter of chronological time. There are inevitable breaks of continuity in any relationship. No practitioner can be available to patients at all times. A good relationship, however, requires continuity of responsibility. Responsible practitioners will provide a deputy who can give care as close as possible to the care they can provide, and they will try to be present at times of great need. We seem almost to have forgotten the importance of presence in medicine. These commitments face us with many conflicting moral choices between obligations to different patients, to our families and to ourselves.

Unconditional commitments sound daunting, and it is true that sticking with a person through thick and thin is hard work. What profession worthy of its name is not demanding? But the general nature of general practice is not as daunting as it is said to be. An openness to any kind of problem does not mean that a GP has to embrace the whole of medical knowledge. GPs have many resources to call on. Even so, the great majority of problems are managed by GPs without outside help, using the traditional methods of listening to patients and performing appropriate examinations. An experienced GP's knowledge includes his or her personal knowledge of patients and their life stories. It is this knowledge, both tacit and explicit, which forms the context for understanding each new problem as it presents, and for designing a plan for management to fit each patient's needs.

The initial assessment

It would be difficult to exaggerate the importance of the initial presentation of illness. How events unfold is profoundly influenced by the doctor's response. In his book, *The Logic of the Sciences and the Humanities*, FSC Northrop wrote: 'The most difficult portion of any inquiry is its initiation. One may have the most rigorous of methods during the later stages of investigation, but if a false or superficial beginning has been made, rigor later on will never retrieve the situation.'[4] The same could be said of the enquiry into a patient's problems. Misdiagnosis of an acute curable condition may result in disability or death. Diagnosis of a spurious disease may set the stage for prolonged invalidism. When ten independent tests are done in healthy people, there is a 40% chance that one will be statistically abnormal and liable to be misinterpreted as evidence of disease.[5] Over-investigation and under-investigation are both potential pitfalls, but general practice has a good record in judicious use of tests.

In the process of diagnosis, the physician interprets the raw data presented by the patient, adds the data acquired by their own search and tries to fit the illness into a disease category within their own frame of reference. In this way, many patients presenting to family physicians have their raw illness differentiated into well-known disease categories. On the other hand, many patients have illnesses that defy this kind of differentiation. There are at least five reasons why this is so:

- An illness may be transient and self-limiting, creating a functional disturbance that clears completely, leaving no evidence on which a diagnosis of disease can be based. These illnesses are usually brief, but not invariably so.
- An illness may be treated so early that it is aborted before it reaches the stage of a definitive diagnosis. Many cases of pneumonia are probably aborted in this way.
- At the edge of every disease category are borderline and intermediate conditions that are difficult or impossible to classify. Because family physicians see all variants of disease, they are likely to encounter milder variants and borderline conditions that may never have been categorised.
- An illness may remain undifferentiated for hours, days or years before its true nature unfolds.
- An illness may be so closely interwoven with the personality and personal life of the patient that it defies classification as a recognisable disease process.

Estimates of how much illness in family practice remains undifferentiated even after assessment vary from 25% to 50%. The exact figure varies with the duration of observation and the criteria adopted for differentiation. Persistently undifferentiated illness has many implications for the clinical method in family practice. The key to its understanding may lie in the patient's life story and relationships, or the doctor–patient relationship, rather than of the disease.

The importance of time in revealing a diagnosis makes clinical observation an important tool in the family physician's hands, and one that he or she has excellent opportunities to use in such instances as segmental pain which eventually reveals itself as herpes zoster, the red circular patch which shows itself to be pityriasis rosea and the persistent cough which is a harbinger of mycoplasma pneumonia.

When patients present their problems, they often do so in a fragmented and oblique manner. There is seldom the neat 'history of present illness' which the conventional clinical method asks us to take. Several problems are often presented at one visit and the most important one for the patient may not be presented first. A patient who presents with a feeling of having a lump in the throat, suggesting globus hystericus, will probably not say that they are afraid it is cancer, but will agree if asked. To reassure them, the doctor has to do a credible examination, check the smoking history and consider whether the patient trusts him enough to accept his reassurance. A patient's deepest hurt, until then unspeakable, may only be revealed when there is complete trust. Even then, they may only be expressed when the patient is leaving (the 'exit problem') or as an aside: 'While I'm here anyway ...'. If there is shame, or fear of rejection, problems may be expressed in indirect rather than in direct language. How illnesses are presented is often recognisably idiosyncratic to a doctor who knows the patient.

Although patients may have their own explanations for their illnesses, it is probably not organised in terms of a medical frame of reference unless they are unusually well informed. Once the patient has been through an assessment process, all this changes. Unless the patient's own frame of reference is very resistant to change, they will tend to see the illness in a different light. Instead of having troublesome pain, the patient will now have a duodenal ulcer. By the direction of the enquiry, the doctor will have taught the patient which symptoms are medically significant and which are not. One cannot observe nature without changing it, a heavy responsibility for the GP. As the first doctor to see the patient, they have great power to change the way the patient perceives and organises the illness. The importance of the initial assessment should make us wary of delegating this task to those with less experience. Minor illness is often a diagnosis made in retrospect.

GPs have to work at all levels of abstraction and all levels of certainty. In the early stages of illness, precise diagnosis may not be possible. This is not because time and resources are lacking, but because the criterial attributes for the diagnosis are not yet present. The early symptoms of life-threatening illnesses, such as meningitis and malaria, are often very similar to those of less serious illnesses. The fact that these are uncommon is no excuse for failure to make an early diagnosis. Sometimes uncertainty can be reduced by safe and simple tests, and there is no excuse for accepting unnecessary levels of uncertainty. Robust 'rule-out' tests with 100% sensitivity are needed to exclude disease that requires early and life-saving treatment. We cannot assume that tests used in other fields are appropriate in primary care. The sensitivity of a test varies with the stage of the illness. A good 'rule-out' test in a fully developed illness may not be sensitive enough in the early stages seen by the family doctor. For example, absence of pyrexia or abdominal tenderness does not rule out appendicitis in the early stages; the heterophil antibody test for infectious mononucleosis is not highly sensitive until the second week of the illness.

On the other hand, the relentless pursuit of certainty can be counter-productive. The predictive value of symptoms and tests varies with the prevalence of the target disorder. A test which has a high predictive value in the selected population of a teaching hospital may have a much lower predictive value in general practice, leading to more false positive results than true positives. The harm done to healthy patients who test positive may outweigh, in the primary care population, the benefits to patients with the target disorder.

How GPs think

I believe it is the attainment of philia[6] – regarded by Aristotle as the highest form of friendship – which accounts for a trait I have noted in GPs: a tendency to concrete rather than abstract thinking. In her interviews with Scottish GPs, Reid[7] observed that some of them 'could not talk about general practice except in terms of their specific patients'. When the conversation is about a disease, we are likely to say 'That reminds me of Mrs X'. This trait is at variance with the abstractive thought which dominates most fields of medicine, especially in the medical school.

Figure 1.1 illustrates the process of abstraction. The three irregular shapes represent patients with similar illnesses. They are all different because no two illnesses are exactly the same. If we are to be healers, we need to know our patients as individuals: they may have their diseases in common, but in their responses to disease, they are unique. The conceptual distinction between illness and disease[8] helps us to understand the process of abstraction. The illness is the patient's experience. The disease is the pathological process doctors use as an explanatory model of the illness, a different perspective on the same reality. The three squares inside the figures represent what the patients have in common. In the process of abstraction we take the common factors and form a disease category: such as multiple, fluctuating neurological symptoms and magnetic resonance imaging (MRI) evidence of demyelination as criteria for multiple sclerosis. Abstraction gives us great predictive power and provides us with our taxonomic language. It enables us to apply our therapeutic technologies with precision. The power of an abstraction depends on its having the same structure as the illness it represents, just as a map has the same structure as a landscape. But it comes at a price. The power of generalisation is gained by distancing ourselves from individual patients and the particulars of their illness. If we look

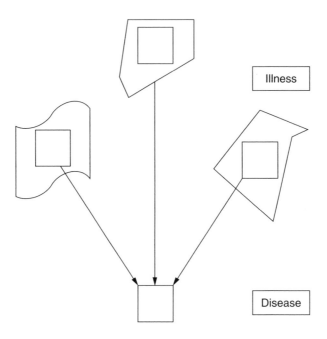

Figure 1.1 The process of abstraction.

Taken from McWhinney IR (2000) Being a general practitioner: what it means. *European Journal of General Practice.* **6** (4): 135–9.

closely, every patient is different in some way. It is in the care of patients that the particulars become crucial.

No abstraction is ever a complete picture of what it represents: it becomes less and less complete as levels of abstraction and power of generalisation increase. Table 1.1 illustrates degrees of abstraction in a patient with multiple, fluctuating neurological symptoms. The first and lowest level is the patient's experience before and after it has been verbalised. Level two is the patient's expressed sensations, feelings and interpretations, and their understanding by the doctor. Level three is the doctor's clinical assessment and analysis of the illness: the clinical diagnosis of multiple sclerosis (MS). Level four is the definitive diagnosis after an MRI scan. As we increase the levels of abstraction, individual differences are ironed out in the interest of generalisation. The lower levels of abstraction are closest to the patient's life world. As we increase the level, the danger is that we forget that our abstraction is not the real world. The diagnosis MS and the MRI scan are not the patient's illness experience. To forget this is, in Alfred Korzybski's[9] aphorism, mistaking the map for the territory.

The ideal is to be capable of both concrete and abstract thinking as required by the occasion. The doctors described by Reid[7] were so concrete in their thinking that they might not be capable of viewing their practice as a population

Table 1.1 Levels of abstraction in a patient with multiple, fluctuating, neurological symptoms and signs

Level 1	Level 2	Level 3	Level 4
Patient's sensations and emotions	Patient's expressed complaints, feelings, interpretations	Doctor's analysis of illness: clinical assessment	MRI scan
Preverbal ↓ verbal	Second-order abstraction	Third-order abstraction	Fourth-order abstraction
'Illness' (patient's experience)	'Illness' (doctor's understanding)	'Disease' (clinical diagnosis: MS)	'Disease' (definitive diagnosis: MS)

Taken from McWhinney IR (1997) *A Textbook of Family Medicine* (2e). Oxford University Press, New York.

at risk. Concrete thinking in its most extreme form may go with a lack of the analytic depth required for precise diagnosis. The neurologist and organismic thinker, Kurt Goldstein, exemplified concrete thinking at its best: he had 'a genius for observing a myriad of minute details combined with the power to see their sense as an organization as a whole'.[10]

Reflecting on her experience as a patient with MS, the philosopher Kay Toombs writes: 'The decisive gap between lived experience and scientific explanation ... is at the root of the fundamental distortion of meaning in the physician–patient relationship.'[11] The distortion results from failure to reconcile the concrete and the abstract. Reaching common ground – one of the key elements of the patient-centred clinical method[12] – is an exchange and synthesis of meanings. The doctor interprets the illness in terms of physical pathology, the name of the disease, causal inferences, prognosis and therapeutic choices. The patient interprets it in terms of experience: what it is like for them, what they believe, fear and expect. Ideally, the exchange results in a synthesis of meanings: they are, after all, perspectives – concrete or abstract – on the same reality. But sometimes a synthesis may not be achieved, at least initially. The doctor's interpretation may be rejected: perhaps the explanation of the patient's chronic pain has been taken to mean that the pain is not 'real'.

Reconciling conflicting perspectives makes some heavy demands on us. It requires us to acknowledge the validity of the patients' experiences and take their interpretation seriously, even if we cannot accept it. We should be aware that our own prejudice, rigidity or faulty logic may be a factor in the disagreement. We may, for example, say that we do not believe in the chronic fatigue syndrome and convey by our body language that we do not believe the patient is sick. We should make sure that doubting patients have all the information we can provide, and have patience as they go through the difficult process of changing their beliefs. And some humility may be called for, as when well informed patients know more than we do about their condition.

Reaching common ground is not a guarantee that it is correct. Both doctor and patient may be wrong about the interpretation of the illness. Sometimes patients have misconceptions which lead them to act against their own interest. It is then the doctor's duty to clarify the issues and place another course of action before the patient, rather than accepting the patient's interpretation without question. This is not the same as failing to respect the patient's autonomy or imposing our own values. There is a long tradition in medicine of a 'therapy of the word', an act of persuasion in which the doctor tries to convince the patient to act in the interest of their health. The act must always take place after the doctor has 'filtered out' any self-interest of their own.[13]

GPs and the human condition

Intimacy with patients brings family doctors face to face with the human condition, especially with human suffering. The experience of suffering looms large in general practice, and we can hardly fail to be deeply aware of the many connections between suffering and illness. The suffering caused by illness is ever present, and there is abundant evidence that grief can cause illness, whether as a trigger, exacerbator or obstacle to healing. It is even possible to die from a broken heart. This is usually referred to as the influence of psychosocial factors in health and disease. But the term psychosocial is an abstraction and strips away the poignancy of what happens. Shakespeare speaks of 'that perilous stuff that weighs upon the heart'.[14] If we speak of suffering we will not be tempted to distance ourselves from the experience. Facing a patient's suffering in this way, not from behind a barrier or as an expert practising a certain technique but as one person to another, is perhaps our most difficult task. But there are rewards, as when we witness the joy of recovery or emergence from despair. Not being tied to a particular disease, organ system or technology makes it easier for us to step out of our abstractions and open ourselves to our patients.

The response to suffering is the essence of healing. Yet to look a patient's suffering in the face without flinching is difficult. It is so easy to withdraw emotionally, to hide behind our abstractions and technologies or, like the priest and the Levite, to avoid the sufferer 'passing by on the other side'. To acknowledge and deal with our disturbing emotions requires self-knowledge. Yet the teaching about the doctor–patient relationship is often 'don't get involved'. In one respect, fear of the emotions is well-founded. To be involved at the level of one's unexamined emotions is potentially harmful. But what the teaching does not say is that involvement is necessary if one is going to be a healer as well as a competent technician. There are right and wrong ways of being involved and this teaching gives no guidance about finding the right way. The teaching is also profoundly mistaken in suggesting that one can encounter suffering and not in some way be affected. Our emotional response may be repressed, but this exacts a heavy price, for repressed emotion may be acted out in ways that are destructive of relationships. There is no such thing as non-involvement and only self-knowledge can protect us from the pitfalls of involvement at the level of our egocentric emotions. Without self-knowledge, moral growth is likely to have shallow roots.

An emblematic case conference

An unusual clinicopathological conference was once held at the Hammersmith Hospital.[15] It was unusual in that the patient's family doctor was present. The subject of the conference was a 50-year-old man with adult coeliac disease, resistant to treatment. Initially, the patient had responded well to a gluten-free diet, but he had later gone downhill very rapidly and died. In opening the discussion, the professor of medicine asked, 'Why did this patient's intestine suddenly become wrecked and remain so wrecked that he died from his disease?'

After a discussion about the pathology of the patient's intestine, the professor commented, 'So it appears that we are completely at sea over the cause of the gut lesion in this man.... the question we have to ask is what would cause it. Dr __, you were this patient's family physician. Would you like to comment ...?'

To this, the patient's family physician replied, 'I would like to suggest that the main reason for this [failure to account for the course of the illness] is the inadequacy of the concepts which they [the discussants] are using in their attempted explanations. If we treat the patient as a biochemical machine and exclude any concepts which refer to him as a person, then it seems to me that explanations of his illness must be extremely limited. If we turn our attention to this man's life pattern and what little we know of his inner feelings, this illness becomes much more understandable ... I know there were major emotional conflicts in all the main areas of his life. The onset of the illness followed the death of his father, an event with which a lot of family feeling was associated. The exacerbation of his illness coincided with rising tension between himself and his adopted daughter within the context of a sterile marriage. The final stage of his illness coincided with the collapse of his work relationship after a long period of devoted service ... I feel that he died because all that he had lived for had somehow come to nothing.'

To this the professor responded, 'Thank you very much. The possibility of a psychogenic influence in coeliac disease has been suggested and clearly if the basic abnormality of coeliac disease is due to a genetically determined enzyme defect, I would find it difficult to believe that psychogenic influences could play much part. It is more likely to be a sensitivity. Do you think that the mucosal lesion was due to an enzyme factor, Dr __?'

This exchange brings to light two seemingly opposite world-views: two different ways of seeing the same reality. We cannot know for certain which was right. But does it really matter? Yes it does. To die unfulfilled is a terrible thing. Surely a doctor caring for such a patient in his last illness should know his condition in all its details. As Cicely Saunders[16] has taught, the pain of the dying is total pain and requires attention to the whole person. Note that the family physician answered the professor's question very precisely. He had not asked 'Why did the patient get coeliac disease?' but 'Why did the patient die?' The family physician shifted the focus from the organ and the disease to the whole person and his life story. There is no contradiction here. If we use 'both/and' instead of 'either/or' thinking, it is possible to die of *both* coeliac disease and a broken heart.

It matters also for other reasons. Hardening of the heart is a very present danger for physicians, and moralists have long drawn attention to those attitudes that harden the heart. Shakespeare's doctor in *Cymbeline*[17] tells the Queen that if she treats living creatures as things, 'Your Highness shall from this practice but make hard your heart'. Literal-mindedness has also been connected with hardness. Two of Dickens' most literal-minded creations, Mr Gradgrind and Ralph Nickleby, are hardness personified. Nickleby pours scorn on the idea that his brother died of a broken heart.

Literal-mindedness has been called the besetting sin of our age.[18] The cardinal virtue – the one that redeems the besetting sin – is imagination, described by Nussbaum[19] as 'the ability to see one thing as another, to see one thing in another'. The literal (utilitarian) mind is 'blind to the qualitative richness of the perceptible world; to the separateness of its people, to their inner depths, their hopes and loves and fears; blind to what it is like to live a human life and to try to endow it with human meaning.'

In a literal-minded, utilitarian age, we are all vulnerable to this blindness and its consequences, though in general practice our openness to patients' experience can help us. Our protection is to keep alive in ourselves the ability to imagine. Without imagination there can be no empathy.

Complexity and the professions

Many of the problems facing the professions in Western countries result from the increasing complexity of human-made systems. In his book, *The Ingenuity Gap*,[20] Thomas Homer-Dixon, a political scientist at the University of Toronto, analyses the critical problems created by the complexity of the modern world. One factor, he writes, is 'the relentless march of technology', with individual new technologies combining to produce unanticipated effects. In medicine, the past decade has seen unprecedented growth in highly effective investigative and therapeutic technologies, together with a revolution in information technology. Homer-Dixon describes six key features of complex systems:

- a large number of parts
- a dense web of causal connections, with multiple feedback loops
- tight coupling and interdependence of components
- openness to their outside environment and indeterminacy of boundaries
- synergy between components
- non-linear behaviour.

In unidirectional systems there are no feedback loops to the system's input. A force acting on a stationary billiard ball has a predictable causal effect. Linear logic is behind many medical procedures and in simple systems can be very effective. The Shouldice Clinic in Toronto repairs hernias using standardised procedures which produce excellent results. The linear logic is appropriate because a hernia is a mechanical defect and can usually be treated as an isolated problem. Many evidence-based guidelines are based on a similar logic and also work well as long as the problem can be isolated, like hypertension in an otherwise healthy and motivated patient. Most chronic diseases, however, are more complex than this. Causes are usually multiple and act together. Co-morbidity is common, making treatment more complicated. For many reasons – mental illness, substance abuse, poverty, overwhelming problems – motivation may be lacking. Patients may be unwilling to change their habits of a lifetime.

According to Homer-Dixon, we have made our social and technological systems so much more complex that we have increased the chance of unexpected destabilising non-linearity. Linear thinking has produced efforts to maximise the benefits of single new technologies, without an understanding of the effects on complex natural systems. As a result, we have antibiotic resistance and the harm done to natural systems by pesticides. 'Our never-ending quest for efficiency, speed and productivity,' says Homer-Dixon, 'causes overspecialization and fragmentation of knowledge, and reduces the availability of general expertise.' He notes that the new communication technologies in financial markets have introduced people with narrow technical and analytical skills, and displaced those with experiential knowledge, which 'consists of intuitions, subtle understandings and finely honed reflexes gained through years of intimate interaction with a given natural, social or technological system.... When we fragment management expertise into subspecialties and squeeze out broad, experiential knowledge, we become more vulnerable to unknown unknowns.'[20] We also make our systems more rigid and less able to respond to crises or adapt to change.

Healthcare is a prime example of an increasingly complex system. In many Western countries this has resulted in an increase in specialisation and a decrease in generalists. Even in systems based on a primary care sector, fragmentation of the generalist role has reduced the comprehensiveness of general practice and in doing so has made it more difficult for GPs to fill their essential role. Applying linear logic, some managed care systems channel patients with chronic diseases into 'silos' where they can receive standardised care from teams of specialised doctors and nurses.

The creation of vertical specialised systems for specific diseases is not new. Up to the 1950s, tuberculosis care had a complete system of clinics, surgical units and sanitoria. When anti-tuberculosis drugs hastened the decline of tuberculosis, the system was completely dismantled. The healthcare system was flexible enough to adapt to the change and tuberculosis physicians found work in the growing fields of respiratory medicine and geriatrics. The tuberculosis subsystem, however, was never completely isolated, and GPs were able to keep in touch with their tuberculosis patients.

Tuberculosis could be a model for silos in the modern system. Cancer and human immunodeficiency (HIV)/AIDS spring to mind as fields that are complex and changing enough to require specialised care over long periods. For patients with HIV/AIDS, it may be a question of moving, by mutual consent, to a GP with more experience in the field. For a high-technology field such as cancer care, the secondary sector is more appropriate, but the silo approach may unintentionally exclude the GP, to the detriment of the patient's overall care.

The alienation of GPs is a potential weakness for any silo or combination of silos. As patients age, co-morbidity increases, and it is likely that a patient will be a member of several silos: perhaps diabetes, cardiac, renal and mental. As the number increases, the difficulties of cross-communication multiply and communication failures occur. In advanced illness, multi-system failure is common, but without generalists, who will coordinate the care? With patients streamed into silos and alienated from their GPs, the relationships we value will be broken and general practice will lose much of its appeal.

Responding to a woman whose husband had received inadequate care for a complex illness, the American surgeon Sherwin Nuland[21] spoke of an essential truth of modern medicine: 'We have trained a generation ... of highly skilled physicians who are inadequate healers. Unable to think of patients as entire human beings, they focus on their own aspects of the problem, and by so much neglect of the complexities of a patient's life ... they make grievous errors ... I have felt ... that specialists are too overwhelmed by what I call "the riddle" of disease to appreciate the totality of human beings' medical care.'

It will not be easy to remedy this situation. A subspecialty requires of the physician intense concentration on a narrow field. It is almost inevitable that specialists will view patients' problems through the lens of their own subject. Where several subspecialists are involved, none of them may feel qualified for the coordinating role. Perhaps we are expecting too much of them. Coordination would more appropriately be provided by the GP, the general internist or the GP with a special interest in internal medicine. Any of these should have the organistic perspective which I believe to be natural for the general practitioner.

The organistic perspective

Since the seventeenth century the dominant Western view of nature has been the mechanistic one, founded on Galilean and Newtonian science, and the philosophy of Bacon and Descartes. The latter's separation of *res extensa* from *res cogitans*, and the reduction of complex phenomena to their simplest components, enabled medicine to make great progress on the assumption that the human body is a machine. The rise of science in seventeenth-century Europe was facilitated by the development of specialised disciplines, each with its own techniques and exclusive focus on the things it did best. The fruits of specialisation were gained by 'narrowing the range of skills that participants were required to master ... (but) the very advantages of disciplinary specialization carried with them the risk that rigour might degenerate into rigidity'.[22]

The discipline of internal medicine arose in the nineteenth century to deal with the complexities of the physiological milieu interior of Claude Bernard and the discoveries of morbid anatomy. Internists were concerned with 'everything under the skin' and by the end of the century had developed a clinical method – differential diagnosis – which used linear logic to connect a patient's illness with anatomical or physiological pathology. With the infectious and deficiency diseases of the nineteenth century the method was very successful. The exemplar of the method was the clinical–pathological conference at which a clinician analysed the evidence and arrived logically at a diagnosis, to be confirmed by the pathologist.

The method has been less successful in some of the dominant diseases of modernity, notably those with a different kind of complexity and little or no anatomical pathology. The human body does have mechanistic features, but a patient is also an organism, and exists in reciprocal relationship with the social and natural environment. If an organism is disturbed or traumatised, the disturbance reverberates throughout the organism. A serious illness affects a person at every level, from the molecular to the cognitive-affective. It is no longer enough to confine our attention to the organs under the skin: we have also to attend to the organism as a whole in relationship with its environment.

By the beginning of the twentieth century, Crookshank[23] observed that textbooks of internal medicine 'gave excellent schemes for the physical examination of the patient, whilst, strangely ignoring almost completely, the psychical (*sic*)'. Since then, modern medicine has divided along a fault line which separates internal medicine, geriatrics and paediatrics from psychiatry, psychogeriatrics and child psychiatry. Each side of the line has its own textbooks and clinical methods. Internal medicine does not attend routinely to the emotions; psychiatry does not require examination of the body, even though psychiatrists prescribe powerful drugs and include bodily disorders such as chronic pain in their practise.

General practice had its origins when apothecaries and surgeons were absorbed into the medical profession during the nineteenth century. Having a different origin and tradition, general practice never divided in this way, and remains the only major discipline which transcends the mind/body fault line. The division is not consistent with the organismic view of the person. Function is an activity of the whole organism. Kurt Goldstein writes, 'Neither does the mind act on the body, nor the body on the mind, no matter how much this may seem to be the case in superficial observation. We are always dealing with the activity of the whole organism, the effects of which refer at one time to something called mind, at another time to something called body.'[24] Goldstein believed that patients as organisms should be analysed in terms of their whole behaviour and interaction with their environment. The human organism has great adaptive powers, enabling it to attain a new kind of wholeness even after devastating losses. But the response to illness is highly individual and to be healers for our patients we have to know them as individuals. Lain Entralgo[25] attributes the failure of Western medicine to integrate the disease with the patient's inner life to the lack, among other things, of a method: 'a technique [for] laying bare, to clinical investigation and to ... pathological consideration, the inner life of the patient ... an exploration method – the dialogue with the patient.' Over the last 50 years, general practice has evolved such a method and it can be adapted to every branch of medicine.

The whole organism is involved in healing. The words whole, health and heal are all derived from the same old English root. Function may be fully restored, or a new but reduced level of wholeness attained by compensation and sub-stitution of other functions, aided by mechanical devices or pharmacological prostheses such as thyroxin. Restoration of function is the aim of physiotherapy, occupation and speech therapy, and of any one who can fill the place of healer in the person's life. Self-assessed function, sense of control and confidence in outcome – all attributes of the whole person – are the best predictors of recovery.[26–28]

The failure to remember that 'mind' and 'body' are abstractions leads to either/or thinking in which diseases are allocated to one or other side of the fault line. A leading neurologist wrote in the *New England Journal of Medicine*: 'Practitioners should recognize that migraine is a neurobiologic, not a psycho-genic disorder.'[29] Why can it not be both? This kind of dualism has long been an obstacle to the integrated approach to patients, leading to dubious concepts such as functional disorders, psychosomatic diseases and somat-isation.[30] By transcending this division, general practice can lead the way towards integration.

The clinical method which has emerged from general practice requires that the whole person (organism) be attended to in every case: the symptoms, the beliefs, the expectations, values and the emotions.[13] The meaning of the illness for the patient is specific for each patient and reflects his or her own unique world.

Specialisation in general practice

Being a generalist should be consistent with having a special field of interest and there has been a growing trend in this kind of specialisation. These practitioners can be consultants for their colleagues and can offer skills such as endoscopy and minor surgery. They can also act as a bridge between primary and secondary sectors – an area in which there are often liaison problems. There are risks involved and we should be aware of the ways in which specialisation could undermine the role of general practice. It is important that GPs with special interests should be firmly rooted in the primary care sector – and still involved in general practice. If they become part of the secondary care sector, they are likely to lose touch with their colleagues in general practice. Having a special interest should not become rigidified into a hierarchical structure in which those who remain full-time generalists are valued less than those with a special interest. Nor should primary care become a mirror image of secondary care, with an array of full-time specialists who have given up general practice and with patients in their field automatically transferred to their care. This would create a silo system in primary care and the logic of having a primary sector would collapse.

Teamwork in general practice

There are two kinds of team. One is assembled for a specific group of patients, such as a family doctor, nutritionist, social worker and psychologist for patients with eating disorders and their families; or, for a patient with diabetes, a family doctor, nurse, diabetologist, nutritionist and chiropodist. Such teams may not work in the same place or meet together regularly, but may need to do so when necessary. The occasion might be a family conference for a patient dying at home. Any member of the team should have the skills to conduct a conference and to lead the team if the main problems are in their field.

The other kind of team is a core group of people who work together day in, day out with the same group of patients, for example one or more GPs, nurses and social workers. The relationships within such a team are crucial. Putting people under one roof does not make them a team. Regular meetings are necessary and some time should be spent in attending to the group process and members' needs. Members of the team should have skills in group relationships and leadership.

The value of teamwork lies in the different perspective that each member brings, resulting in mutual enlightenment and an increment of patient care. If there is no value added for the patient, it is not a well-functioning team. Although there is some overlap of roles, each member has a central role that is recognised by the group. Whoever is leading the team should make clear who is responsible for implementing decisions reached about patient care, thus avoiding the confusion of responsibility which is a risk of teamwork. If a team is well led and meets regularly, the special perspective of each member should soon be recognised. Changes in a member's role in patient care may require adjustments by other members.

A key issue for primary care teams is the initial assessment of patients and the changing role of nurses. According to one school of thought, patients should be assessed first by a nurse, who deals with minor illnesses and directs other patients to the appropriate member of the team. This has the potential for causing problems both for nursing and medicine. If the overlap is small, and the nurse functions as a physician's assistant, the role may become a subprofessional one, and the team may lose the benefit of a nursing perspective. On the other hand, if the overlap is large, nurse practitioners may replace physicians and are likely to be reclassified as physicians at some future time. This is what happened in the nineteenth century when apothecaries became defined as medical practitioners. Other professionals have much to learn from nursing's unique approach to patient care, and it is important that this is not lost as nurses move into new roles. Besides the nurses who are members of the primary care team, others who have special skills in fields such as asthma, diabetes and colostomy care have so much to offer patients and to teach us. For medical practitioners, clinical diagnosis is a central role and years of medical education are devoted to developing the skills. It may be argued that relieving doctors of minor illness leaves them more time to spend with difficult diagnostic problems, but this does not take account of the difficulty of defining minor illness. Reducing the number of initial assessments that GPs do on their own patients could reduce the knowledge of patients that accumulates over the years, and make them less skilful in the assessment of undifferentiated illnesses. A GP might become a doctor, who, when asked if they have seen Mrs X says, 'Oh yes, you mean the systemic lupus'. Moreover, any rigid system which denies direct access of patients to their doctors is not patient-centred. Patients may develop relationships with any member of the team and should be in a position to decide which member will meet their need. Finally, let us not forget the relationship-building value of all consultations, however minor. A minor consultation can still be the occasion for small courtesies that are so important in the cultivation of friendship. The more these common courtesies can become habits, the more secure the virtues of friendliness will be, and the less vulnerable to the stresses and difficulties of medical practice.[31]

The way ahead

Provided we ourselves remain true to the essence of general practice, we have nothing to fear from change. Whatever else changes, there will always be suffering and there will always be people who are yearning for healing. There will always be people who are looking for the kind of commitment we can offer. Our greatest challenges will be not only keeping up to date with technical advances, but preparing ourselves to be healers. This will mean cultivating our openness to patients and colleagues; learning to listen with total attention, as Michael Balint[32] described and exemplified; and mastering the skills of relationship – skills which require personal change in ourselves and the ability to examine our own perspectives, motives and beliefs. As I meet GPs from many parts of the world, I am impressed by how many of them are going through this process. In the long run it may be our greatest contribution to medicine.

Acknowledgements

My thanks are due to the people who reviewed previous drafts of this chapter and gave me thoughtful comments and suggestions: Michael Atkinson, Tom Freeman, Ann Louise Kinmonth, Betty McWhinney, Heather McWhinney and Joe Morrissy: also to Joanna Llorca Asuncion for preparing successive drafts of the manuscript.

References

1   Popper KR (1972) *Conjectures and Refutations: the growth of scientific knowledge*. Routledge, Paul Kegan, London.

2   Hjortdahl P (1992) Continuity of care: general practitioners' knowledge about, and sense of responsibility towards, their patients. *Family Practice.* **9**: 3.

3   McWhinney IR (1997) *A Textbook of Family Medicine*, pp. 187–9. Oxford University Press, New York.

4   Northrop FSC (1959) *The Logic of the Sciences and the Humanities*. Meridian Books, The World Publishing Company, Cleveland, Ohio.

5   Galen RS and Gambino SR (1975) *Beyond Normality: the predictive value and efficiency of medical diagnoses*. John Wiley, New York.

6   Toulmin SE (2001) *Return to Reason*, p. 34. Harvard University Press, Cambridge, MA.

7   Reid M (1982) Marginal man: the identity dilemma of the academic general practitioner. *Symbolic Interaction.* **5** (2): 325.

8   Fabrega H (1974) *Disease and Social Behavior.* MIT Press, Cambridge, MA.

9   Korzybski A (1958) *Science and Sanity: an introduction to non-Aristotelian systems and general semantics* (4e). International Non-Aristotelian Library Publishing Co., Lake Bille, CT.

10   Sacks O (2000) Foreword to: Goldstein K *The Organism: a holistic approach to biology derived from pathological data in man.* Zone Books, New York.

11 Toombs SK (1995) *The Meaning of Illness: a phenomenological account of the different perspectives of physician and patient.* Kluwer, Dordrecht.

12 Stewart MA, Brown JB, Weston WW *et al.* (1995) *Patient-centered Medicine: transforming the clinical method.* Sage, Newbury Park, CA.

13 Nussbaum MC (1995) *Poetic Justice: the literary imagination and public life*, p. 74. Beacon Press, Boston, MA.

14 Shakespeare W *Macbeth*, Act IV, Scene III.

15 Clinicopathological Conference (1968) A case of adult coeliac disease resistant to treatment. *BMJ.* **1**: 678.

16 Saunders C (1984) The philosophy of terminal care. In: Saunders C (ed) *The Management of Terminal Malignant Disease* (2e). Edward Arnold, London.

17 Shakespeare W *Cymbeline*, Act I, Scene V.

18 Barfield O (1957) *Saving the Appearances: a study in Idolatry.* Faber and Faber, New York.

19 Nussbaum MC (1995) *Poetic Justice: the literary imagination and public life*, pp. 26–7. Beacon Press, Boston, MA.

20 Homer-Dixon T (2001) *The Ingenuity Gap.* Vintage Canada, Toronto.

21 Nuland S (2002) 'Complications': an exchange. *The New York Review of Books.* Y.XLIX, Number 20, pp. 88–9.

22 Toulmin SE (2001) *Return to Reason*, p. 41. Harvard University Press, Cambridge, MA.

23 Crookshank FG (1926) The Theory of Diagnosis. *Lancet.* **2**: 939.

24 Goldstein K (1939) *The Organism: a holistic approach to biology derived from pathological data in man*, pp. 264–5. Zone Books, New York.

25 Entralgo PL (1956) *Mind and Body.* PJ Kennedy, New York.

26 Idler EL (1992) Self-assessed health and mortality: a review of studies. In: Maes S, Leventhal H and Johnston M (eds) *International Review of Health Psychology.* John Wiley, New York.

27 Siegrist J (1993) Sense of coherence and sociology of emotion. Comment on Antonovsky. *Social Science and Medicine.* **37**: 974.

28 Sobel DS (1995) Rethinking medicine: improving health outcomes with cost-effective psychosocial interventions. *Psychosomatic Medicine.* **57**: 234.

29 Olesen J (1994) Understanding the biological basis of migraine. *New England Journal of Medicine.* **331**: 1713–14.

30 McWhinney IR, Epstein RM and Freeman TR (2001) Somatization – 'medicine's unsolved problem'. *Advances in Mind–Body Medicine.* **17** (4): 232–9.

31 Drane JF (1995) *Becoming a Good Doctor: the place of virtue and character in medical ethics* (2e). Speed and Ward, Kansas City.

32 McWhinney IR (1999) Fifty years on: the legacy of Michael Balint. *British Journal of General Practice.* **49**: 418–19.

CHAPTER 2

The effectiveness of primary healthcare

Barbara Starfield

Throughout the world, primary care is considered to be the basic level of health-care provision. Despite the near-universal agreement of the importance of primary care, the concept of 'general practice' is increasingly threatened by interests vested in the technological aspects of medical care generally associated with subspecialism. The purpose of this chapter is to highlight the special contributions made by primary care within health services systems and to suggest that a continued focus on primary care will be necessary for further progress in improving both average levels of health as well as its distribution in populations.

The generally poor relationship between the physician/population ratio and health of populations, at least in industrialised nations, has been recognised for decades. In many studies, greater ratios have been associated with *worse* health levels; mortality rates have been noticed to fall when physicians go on strike. It is common wisdom that medical care contributes relatively little to improved health rates when examined historically; public health and social advances are thought to contribute more. The best information on the relative benefit from personal health services is that they have contributed about half of the im-provement in life expectancy, at least in the UK and in the United States (US).[1] To date, no one has systematically explored the extent to which primary care, as a major component of personal health services, contributes to this effect.

Contributions to health made by personal health services fit into several categories: prevention, morbidity, life expectancy and mortality, and equity in the distribution within and across populations on each of these characteristics. In addition, there are the important policy-relevant considerations of demand on society's resources in the form of hospitalisations and costs of care.

Box 2.1 provides a parsimonious list of indicators that should be responsive to primary care, at least according to a series of informal focus groups of pri-mary care 'experts' in the US and elsewhere. The following sections present the

---

Box 2.1 Indicators for evaluating primary care at population levels

- Accomplishments in prevention not related to specific diseases: immunisation status; personal health behaviours (breastfeeding, not smoking, use of seat-belts, use of smoke detectors, physical activity, good diet)
- Unwanted pregnancies
- Low incidence of vaccine-preventable diseases
- Early detection of risk for child abuse
- Low incidence of attempted suicide
- Low incidence of accidental poisoning
- Improved quality of life, including decreased disability from:
  - asthma
  - osteoarthritis
  - post-myocardial infarct
- Shortened duration of symptoms associated with peptic ulcers
- Reduced use of unnecessary resources, including:
  - laboratory tests and procedures
  - unjustified medications (such as antibiotics for influenza, growth hormone treatment for short children)
- Low incidence of adverse effects of medications
- Reduced frequency of conditions related to prevention: stroke, amputations resulting from diabetes complications, surgery for preventable eye conditions, incidence of sexually transmitted diseases and AIDS
- Low post-neonatal mortality rates
- Improved quality of dying/terminal care
- Rates of death due to:
  - asthma
  - hypertensive and cerebrovascular disease
- Hospitalisations for ambulatory care-sensitive conditions
- For all health indicators: reductions in disparities across population subgroups

---

basis for hypothesising that primary care would contribute especially to health in these areas and evidence for its benefits to the health of the population in each of these areas. The preponderance of evidence for the value of primary care comes from the US, for the reason that primary care appears to be more under attack and more questioned than is the case in many other countries that accept primary care at face value.

The evidence provided is conservative in that the requirements for specification of primary care were strict. Not included is the large amount of detailed evidence that access to health services makes a difference to health status as measured in various ways,[1,2] or evidence that association with a 'regular' or 'usual' source of care also has positive impacts (e.g. Starfield[3]). Such considerations are most important in the US, where access to care is not universal, and where access, even if present, is not necessarily with a primary care physician. Moreover, evidence was sought from sources that examined primary care as a whole, rather than specific aspects of primary care (such as continuity of care, comprehensiveness of care or coordination of care). (For evidence of the benefits of each of these components of primary care, *see* Starfield.[4]) There is also considerable and consistent evidence that primary care physicians are much more likely to achieve cardinal primary care practice characteristics that are themselves known to improve health.[5,6]

Why *should* primary care contribute to better health? There is good theory as to why primary care should have an effect, and on what aspects of health. The following sections review the rationale and the evidence in these different categories.

Primary prevention

Whereas preventive interventions might be better performed by specialists if the interventions are in the specialists' area of expertise, it is in primary care that preventive interventions not related to any one disease or organ system should be best carried out. Thus, for example, rates of cholesterol testing might be highest in the practices of cardiologists (who are more likely to follow patients with cardiovascular disease). However, immunisations and encouragement of healthy personal behaviour should be best carried out by primary care physicians because these types of physicians focus on persons rather than diseases, and because their practices follow a more general cross-section of the population. Examples of these 'generic' personal health behaviours include breastfeeding, no smoking, use of seat-belts, use of smoke detectors, physical activity and healthy diets. Evidence confirms these hypotheses. US states with higher ratios of primary care physicians to population have lower smoking rates, less obesity and higher seat-belt use than states with lower primary care to population ratios.[7,8] Continuity of care with a *single* provider was positively associated with primary preventive care, including smoking cessation and influenza immunisation, in a large ongoing 60-community study in the US.[9] Population subgroups with a good primary care source have better birth weight distributions than comparable populations without good primary care. In both white and African-American populations in both urban and rural areas in the US, rates of low birth weight are lower where the source of care is a community health centre designed to provide good primary care than in the comparable population as a whole.[10] The likelihood of having any preventive visits among disadvantaged children is much greater when their source of care is a good primary care practitioner.[11]

Secondary prevention

To the extent that most secondary preventive activities are disease focused, better quality for primary care (as compared with speciality care) would not necessarily be expected. However, the evidence suggests otherwise for those conditions that are common and hence in the province primarily of primary care. Another large study of differences between primary care physicians and specialists caring for patients with hypertension, non-insulin-dependent diabetes, recent myocardial infarction or depression showed that the only preventive care procedures better performed by specialists were checks for foot-ulcer and infection status among patients of endocrinologists.[12] Moreover, approaches to prevention in primary care practice (general practice) are more generic and result in more improvement in patients' health status than is the case in speciality-oriented practice.[13] When data are obtained from the general community rather than from practices, having a good primary care source is the major determinant of receiving even disease-focused preventive care consisting of blood pressure screening, clinical breast exams, mammograms and Pap (cervical) smears.[14]

Disease management

Following the line of reasoning established above, it might be expected that specialists would perform better than generalists and achieve better outcomes for those conditions within their purview. For example, gastroenterologists adopted antibiotic therapy earlier than did generalists (except if the generalists worked in groups with gastroenterologists).[15] That this is the case has been demonstrated repeatedly in studies designed by specialists to compare the quality of care in speciality practice and in generalist practice.[16] Most studies that compare generalists and specialists conclude that condition-specific quality of care provided by specialists is better when the condition is in their area of special interest, using indicators of quality of care such as the performance of indicated preventive procedures, the performance of indicated laboratory tests for monitoring disease status, the prescribing of indicated medications[17] and in adherence to guidelines. The few studies planned and executed by generalists[18,19] conclude that quality of care is the same or that primary care is better, suggesting possible differences in conceptualisation of appropriate 'outcomes' by the two types of physicians, with specialists more concerned with specific disease-related measures. Few studies have examined generic outcomes in terms of health status or quality of care *other* than for the particular conditions under study, even though evidence indicates that co-morbidity engenders more visits to both generalists and specialists than does the index condition.[20] If it is patient health (rather than disease processes or outcomes) that is of interest as the proper focus of health services, primary care programmes clearly provide superior care, especially for conditions that are commonly seen in primary care. An elegant case–control study[21] categorised men appearing at an emergency room in a large metropolitan area as having complications of hypertension or as having another condition while incidentally having hypertension that was uncomplicated. Those with complications of hypertension were much less likely to have a source of primary care than men whose hypertension was an incidental finding. The presence of a source of primary care was the most notable and significant finding between the two groups.

In another demonstration of the effectiveness of primary care even for disease-oriented care, GP diabetic clinics in the UK were found to do as well as hospital specialists in monitoring for diabetic complications.[22] It should also be noted that in systems where the GPs are educated and have an organised system for recall, GP care for diabetic patients yields better results than those of specialists in hospitals. In such situations, patients of GPs have lower mortality and better glycaemic control than is the case for patients treated in hospitals.[23]

Rates of complications, readmission to hospital and length of convalescence are the same after early discharge from the hospital after minor surgery, regardless of whether the care was provided by the hospital outpatient department or GPs.[24]

Thus, even when considering care for many specific common diseases, primary care physicians perform at least as well as specialists. (For uncommon conditions, appropriate specialist care is undoubtedly better as primary care physicians would not see them frequently enough to maintain competence in managing them.)

Hospitalisations and emergency care use

The literature is strong in showing that lower rates of hospitalisation for ambulatory care-sensitive conditions (hospitalisations that should be prevented with good primary care) are strongly associated with receipt of primary care. Geographic areas with more family and general practitioners have lower hospitalisation rates for these types of conditions, including diabetes mellitus or pneumonia in children and five adult conditions (angina, congestive heart failure, hypertension, pneumonia, diabetes mellitus).[25] Children receiving their care from a good primary care source have lower hospitalisation rates for these conditions as well as a lower hospitalisation rate overall; these findings are associated with the better receipt of preventive care (*see* above) received from primary care providers.[11] Rates of hospital admission are lower in US communities in which primary care physicians are more involved in the care of children both before and during hospitalisation.[26] Adolescents with the same regular source of care for preventive and illness care (that is, a source of primary care) are much more likely to receive indicated preventive care and less likely to seek care in emergency rooms.[27]

In the UK, a study showed the high salience of primary care for in-hospital mortality; the primary care physician supply was more powerfully associated with reductions in in-hospital standardised mortality than the number of doctors per 100 hospital beds.[28] A later study showed that, after controlling for social class, deprivation index, ethnicity and limiting long-term illness, each unit increase in GP supply per 10 000 population was significantly associated with a decrease in hospital admission rates of about 14 per 100 000 for acute illnesses and about 11 per 100 000 for chronic illnesses.[29]

Thus, there is strong and consistent evidence that hospitalisations, and especially hospitalisations for ambulatory care-sensitive conditions, are less frequent when primary care is strong.

Costs of care

Areas in which primary care is stronger, as measured by primary care physician to population ratios, have much lower total healthcare costs than other areas. This has been demonstrated to be the case among the elderly in the US who live in metropolitan areas for both total costs (inpatient and outpatient)[30,31] and for the total population in the US,[32] as well as in an international comparison of industrialised countries.[33] Care for illnesses common in the population, e.g. community-acquired pneumonia, is more expensive if provided by specialists than if provided by generalists, with no difference in outcomes.[34,35]

Morbidity

Primary care physician supply has been demonstrated to be related to lower rates of reporting poor or fair health in 60 representative US communities, after controlling for a wide variety of characteristics also known to be related to self-reported health (in particular, a range of socio-demographic and socio-economic characteristics).[36] Data from this same survey confirmed the positive impact of primary care by showing that those who actually experienced better primary care reported better health. Receiving good primary care accounted for greater than a 5% reduction in reporting of poor health and a 6% reduction in reporting of depression. Those with the best quality of primary care showed an 8% reduction in reporting of poor health and more than 10% reduction in reporting feeling depressed.[37] Outcomes of care after surgery in Canada have also been shown to be better when primary care physicians referred children to specialists for recurrent tonsillitis or otitis media, as compared with referral by a specialist.[38] The children had fewer postoperative complications, a greater decrease in respiratory episodes following surgery and a greater decrease in episodes of otitis media after surgery.

Birth weight (and infant mortality) were also associated with primary care physician supply in US states. A pooled, cross-sectional, time-series analysis of 11 years (1985–95) of state-level (US) data showed that the higher the primary care physician supply, the lower the low birth weight percentage and the lower the infant mortality, even after controlling for educational levels, unemployment, racial/ethnic composition, income inequality and urban–rural differences.[39]

One population-based study[40] in an entire US state found that detection of colorectal cancer at earlier stages was better in areas that had a greater supply of primary care physicians. Conversely, diagnosis tended to be later in areas with more specialist physicians. The nature of the findings led the authors to conclude that a lower supply of specialists enhances the likelihood that primary care physicians screen for such cancers.

Mortality

Perhaps the most frequent demonstration of the benefits of primary care has been with regard to mortality. One line of evidence comes from ecological studies of the relationship between primary care personnel to population ratios and various types of health outcomes in the US. Two separate studies found better health outcomes in states with higher primary care/physician ratios after controlling for socio-demographic measures (% elderly, % urban, % minority, education, income, unemployment, pollution) and lifestyle factors (seat-belt use, obesity and smoking). These studies operationalised primary care as physicians in family practice and general practice, general internal medicine and general paediatrics.[7,41,42] The outcomes included overall mortality, mortality from heart disease, mortality from cancer, neonatal mortality, life span and low birth weight.

Adding to this cross-sectional evidence are the findings of a longitudinal analysis of state-level data on total mortality from 1985 to 1995, while controlling for ethnicity, unemployment, education and income inequality. The analysis showed that an increase of one primary care physician per 10 000 population is associated with a reduction of 144 deaths per 100 000 population. In addition to a contemporaneous effect, primary care also has an increasing, latent effect in reducing mortality.[43]

Similar evidence from Spain showed the effect of primary care reform on mortality rates for several major causes of death.[44] The researchers divided Barcelona into zones based on how early primary reform was implemented. Theory about the impact of primary care would suggest that deaths associated with hypertension and stroke would be responsive to primary care alone, whereas deaths from perinatal causes, cervical cancer and cirrhosis would also require improvements in speciality care for mortality to be reduced. Ten years after the reform was implemented, death rates associated with hypertension and stroke fell the most in those zones in which reform was implemented. Even lung cancer deaths increased less in areas with primary care reform than in other areas. For perinatal causes, death rates fell, but not more in the zones with earlier primary care reform. The same was the case for deaths associated with cervical cancer and cirrhosis. For tuberculosis, rates in all three zones decreased, consistent with a city-wide public health campaign to address the problem.

A pooled, cross-sectional, time-series analysis of 11 years of state-level (US) data showed that primary care physician supply was related to lower rates of stroke mortality, even after controlling for income inequality, education levels, unemployment, racial/ethnic composition and rural–urban distribution, thus confirming the Barcelona finding regarding the association of primary care with deaths associated with effects of hypertension.[45]

The second line of evidence comes from studies with the individual as the unit of analysis. A nationally representative survey showed that adult US respondents who reported a primary care physician rather than a specialist as their regular source of care had lower subsequent five-year mortality, after controlling for initial differences in health status, demographic characteristics, health insurance status, health perceptions, reported diagnoses and smoking status.[32]

The same is the case when the analyses addressed premature mortality (mortality before age 75), at least in US metropolitan areas, even when a large number of other possible influences, including characteristics of the communities, are taken into account. (In rural areas of the US, the supply of physicians is relatively much less and much more variable, so that the effect of primary care is not found.[46])

Figure 2.1 shows the positive association between life expectancy and more primary care physicians in the 50 US states. The greater the ratio of physicians per population, the greater the life expectancy.[8] Even greater precision in estimation of the benefits of primary care comes from two more recent studies in US states and metropolitan areas in which the possible mitigating effects of income inequality were added to path analyses.[8,47] Both less income inequality and primary care physician availability were found to be independently associated with better health as measured by a variety of common health indicators. However, they differed in their effect in that income inequality was particularly associated with percentage of infants born at low birth weight and with total neonatal mortality. In contrast, primary care physician availability was particularly associated with lower mortality from stroke and the post-neonatal component of infant mortality. Both have a major impact on total mortality and life expectancy,[8] but neither has an effect on cancer mortality. Income inequality also has an indirect effect through primary care, such that areas that are more highly income equitable are also likely to have better primary care physician to population ratios. While the effect of income inequality is approximately the same in African-American populations as in white populations, the effect of primary care is less in the former, possibly because the mere presence of primary care physicians may not reflect the actual availability of these physicians to African-American populations in the US.[47]

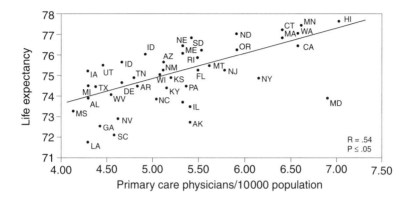

Figure 2.1 State level analysis: primary care physicians/population positively associated with longer life expectancy.[41]

Equity

Primary care has been shown to reduce disparities in health. For example, higher primary care physician to population ratios are associated with greater effects in areas of high income inequality, at least for post-neonatal mortality, stroke mortality and self-reported health. Areas with high primary care resources and high income inequality had 17% lower post-neonatal mortality (compared with the population mean) whereas post-neonatal mortality in similar high inequality areas but low primary care resources was 7% higher. For stroke mortality, the comparable figures were 2% lower mortality where primary care resources were high and 1% higher where the primary care resources were low. The figures were even more striking in the case of self-reported health, where high income inequality areas were 33% higher in reporting of fair or poor health if primary care resources were low (calculated from data in Shi and Starfield[36]).

A related study found a relationship between primary care and reduction of disparities in self-reported health and in self-perceived depression between more advantaged and less advantaged communities in the US. After controlling for the socio-demographic characteristics of age, race/ethnicity, education, employment status and type, quartiles of family income, health insurance and smoking, people's experiences with primary care were found to be significantly related to reported good health as well as less depression. In contrast to prior studies in which primary care was assessed by primary care to population ratios, this study demonstrated the relationship at the individual level between better primary care experiences and better health.[37] Good primary care experiences were able to reduce the adverse effect of income inequality on health as disparities in self-rated health between higher and lower income inequality areas were reduced where primary care experiences were stronger.

In the longitudinal US study of total mortality mentioned above, the association between higher primary care physician supply and lower mortality was greater in the African-American population than in the white majority population, indicating a reduction in racial disparities in mortality.[43]

Studies in developing countries show the same benefit from primary care as compared with overall benefit from health services. In seven African countries, the highest 20% of the population receives well over twice as much financial benefit from overall government spending (40% versus 12%). But for primary care services, the poor–rich ratio is notably lower (23% versus 15%),[48] leading one expert to conclude that, from an equity perspective, 'the move toward primary care represents a clear step in the right direction'.[49]

An unusual demonstration of the likely effect of primary care found that African-Americans in London have no greater rates of diabetes-related lower-extremity amputation[50] whereas African-Americans in the US have rates two to three times that of the white population. In men, the rates were lower in the African-American men than in the white population, a difference wholly accounted for by lower rates of smoking, neuropathy and peripheral vascular disease. The findings persisted even after control for socio-economic differences. In the UK, of course, there is ready access to a source of primary care for everyone, whereas this is not the case in the US where the 'safety net' is often a place such as many hospital outpatient departments, which are not organised to provide the basic elements of primary care.

International comparisons

There has been increasing evidence associating primary care with improved health outcomes in international comparison studies. The first such evidence derives from an ecological study conducted in 11 Western industrialised countries.[51,52] In this study, the strength of the primary care infrastructure was characterised by scoring five characteristics of the health system that are considered conducive to a strong primary care infrastructure (including primary care physician/population ratios), and six characteristics of people's experiences in receiving care that are generally considered to reflect strong primary care. The first point to be made is that the score for practice characteristics follows the score for system characteristics. That is, an adequate delivery of services requires adequate governmental policies. The second point is that those countries with weak primary care infrastructures had higher costs and poorer outcomes, most especially notable in those indicators in early childhood where the greatest impact of primary care services to women and children would be expected: low birth weight and post-neonatal mortality. A more recent comparison, with 13 countries and an expanded set of indicators of both primary care and health outcomes, had similar findings. In particular, the stronger the primary care, the lower the costs. Countries with weak primary care infrastructures have poorer performance on most major aspects of health. In contrast, countries with the strongest primary care infrastructures have better health on just those aspects of health that are most amenable to primary care: post-neonatal mortality and years of potential life lost due to suicide. Low birth weight rates are also lowest in these countries, possibly due to a beneficial effect of primary care on mothers' health *before* pregnancy.[33] The most salient characteristics of primary care and policy-related determinants of primary care orientation were degree of comprehensiveness and family orientation, and government attempts to distribute resources equitably, publicly accountable universal financial coverage and low or no cost sharing for primary care services.[33] The latter two have been studied and confirmed by Or.[53]

Macinko *et al.*[54] recently supported these conclusions in a much more extensive time-series analysis across 19 Organisation for Economic Cooperation and Development (OECD) countries. The stronger the primary care orientation of the country, the lower the all-cause mortality, all-cause premature mortality and cause-specific premature mortality from asthma and bronchitis, emphysema and pneumonia, cardiovascular disease and heart disease. The relationship was robust even after controlling for a variety of macro-level characteristics (gross domestic product [GDP] per capita, total physicians per 1000 population, percentage of elderly people) and micro-level characteristics (average number of ambulatory care visits, per capita income, alcohol and tobacco consumption). It was estimated that improving a country's primary care score by five points (on a 20-point scale) could reduce premature deaths for pneumonia and influenza, and asthma and bronchitis by as much as 50%; reduction in premature mortality for cerebrovascular and heart disease could be as high as 25%.

Primary care in the future

What issues remain to be addressed in primary care to enhance its contribution to health of populations and equity in distribution of health?

The greatest challenges to primary care concern adequate recognition and management of co-morbidity, preventing the adverse effects of medical interventions, maintaining high quality of the important characteristics of primary care practice and addressing the need to improve equity in health services and in health of populations.[55]

Co-morbidity is a major challenge. Historically, principles of delivery of medical care have been based on the prevention and management of specific diseases. In the current climate of evidence-based medicine, guidelines for the management of diseases are proliferating and increasingly used. The development of guidelines is generally based on evidence from the literature that certain modes of management achieve better outcomes than others. The 'gold standard' for evidence is the randomised controlled clinical trial, which excludes, as a criterion for participation in the trial, individuals with co-morbid conditions. Co-morbidity (the simultaneous presence of apparently unrelated conditions) is common in the population and not randomly distributed. Although co-morbidity increases in frequency with age, it is in the young that co-morbidity occurs much more frequently than expected by chance occurrence of two or more conditions.[56] Data systems should be developed that provide a much better basis for examining the distribution and nature of co-morbidity in primary care; ascertainment of evidence on the impact of co-morbidity on responsiveness to medical interventions will be needed if primary care practice is to be made more appropriately evidence based.

Primary care practitioners are in the best position to detect the occurrence of potential adverse effects of medical interventions, particularly those stemming from drug reactions and interactions. In systems of care that are oriented to primary care (including some Health Maintenance Organizations [HMOs] in the United States), primary care practitioners are, by far, the most commonly seen physician for patients with *all* degrees of co-morbidity, and both for single common conditions *and* for co-morbid conditions. Only when individual conditions are uncommon are specialists the most frequent type of physician seen, and only for that condition (*not* for co-morbid conditions).[20] Thus, primary care physicians are more likely to see the adverse events that result from their own care as well as the care of others whom the patient may see. The challenge for primary care is to develop systems to code presenting symptoms or signs that are unexpected, and to develop information systems that could serve as early warnings of the occurrence of systematic adverse events in persons previously subjected to particular types of interventions. It is possible that the International Classification of Primary Care (ICPC)[57] could serve as the basis for recording and classifying these symptoms and signs.

Primary care is also faced with imperatives to continuously improve not only the clinical quality of its services but also its mode of delivery with respect to the cardinal features of primary care practice: first contact care, ongoing person-focused care over time, comprehensiveness of services and coordination of care, as well as features of care that derive from high levels of performance of the cardinal features (family-centredness, community orientation and cultural competence).[4]

First contact care means that people should consult the primary care practitioners rather than someone else the first time they perceive a new need for care.

Ongoing person-focused care means that care should be focused on the person rather than on the disease; at least two years of a relationship (and as many as five) are generally required for patients and practitioners to know each other well enough to provide optimum person-focused care. A freely chosen primary care practitioner provides better assurance that a good relationship will be achieved than is the case if the practitioner is assigned.

Evidence is strong on the benefits of an ongoing relationship with a particular provider rather than with a particular place or no place at all. People with no source of primary care are more likely to be hospitalised, to delay in receiving needed and timely preventive care, to receive care in emergency departments, to have higher subsequent mortality and higher healthcare costs, and less likely to see a physician in the presence of symptoms. People with just a place (such as a particular hospital clinic) are somewhat better off, in that they are more likely to keep their appointments, have fewer hospitalisations and lower costs, and receive generally better preventive care. Many studies show, however, that people who report a particular doctor as their regular source of care receive more appropriate preventive care, have their problems better recognised, have fewer diagnostic tests and fewer prescriptions, have fewer hospitalisations and visits to emergency departments, and are more likely to have more accurate diagnoses and lower costs of care. Table 2.1 summarises the strength of the evidence on these benefits of an ongoing relationship.

Comprehensiveness means that all problems in the population should be cared for in primary care (with short-term referral as needed) except those that are too uncommon (generally a frequency of less than one or two per 1000 in the population served) for the primary care practitioner or team to maintain competence in dealing with them.

Coordination of care means that the primary care practice must integrate all aspects of care when patients must be seen elsewhere. As 13–20% of an average practice population will require referral in a year, this burden is considerable. Very few health systems, even those that are considered to rate high on primary

Table 2.1 Benefits of longitudinality, based on evidence from the literature

	Identification with a person	Identification with a place
Better problem/needs recognition	++	
More accurate/earlier diagnosis	++	
Better concordance		
Appointment keeping	++	++
Treatment advice	++	
Less emergency room use	++	
Fewer hospitalisations	++	+
Lower costs	++	+
Better prevention (some types)	++	++
Better monitoring	+	
Fewer drug prescriptions	+	
Increased satisfaction	++	

++ Evidence good
 + Evidence moderate

care, achieve high levels of coordination of care, at least as measured by transfer of information from primary care physicians to specialists, and vice versa. The challenge for primary care is to develop systems to facilitate coordinating efforts.[4]

It is likely that better coordination of care – itself a result of the better systems of care in which physicians work – is responsible for whatever benefits well-organised HMOs in the US have over general health systems, even those in countries that are highly primary care oriented. For example, and despite design limitations of the study comparing the Kaiser–Permanente healthcare plan in the US with the National Health Service (NHS) in the UK,[58] the lower hospitalisation rates and lower resource use in the former may well be a result of a system specifically designed to enhance coordination between primary care physicians and specialists.

Finally, the achievement of equity in health services and health is an imperative everywhere. Primary care is inherently a more equitable level of care than other levels of care. It is least costly (hence sparing resources that could be devoted to equalising health services benefits to more disadvantaged populations);[4] through its cardinal features it achieves better outcomes for populations. The extent to which primary care in fact does achieve better equity depends on the provision of information by health authorities as to the needs in the various areas on which primary care practices are located. Better computerised information systems, both at the area level, and at the practice level, will help enhance the already strong benefits of primary care to the health of individuals, population subgroups and populations.

Supported in part by Grant No. 6 U30 CS 00189-05 S1 R1 of the Bureau of Primary Health Care, Health Resources and Services Administration, Department of Health and Human Services, to the Primary Care Policy Center for the Undeserved at Johns Hopkins University.

References

1 Bunker J (2001) *Medicine Matters After All: measuring the benefits of medical care, a healthy lifestyle and a just social environment.* Nuffield Trust, London.

2 Starfield B (1985) *The Effectiveness of Medical Care: validating clinical wisdom.* Johns Hopkins University Press, Baltimore, MD.

3 Starfield B (2000) Evaluating the State Children's Health Insurance Program: critical considerations. *Annual Review of Public Health.* **21**: 569–85.

4 Starfield B (1998) *Primary Care: balancing health needs, services, and technology.* Oxford University Press, New York.

5 Weiner JP and Starfield B (1983) Measurement of the primary care roles of office-based physicians. *American Journal of Public Health.* **73**: 666–71.

6   Rosenblatt RA, Hart LG, Baldwin LM *et al.* (1998) The generalist role of specialty physicians: is there a hidden system of primary care? *Journal of the American Medical Association.* **279**: 1364–70.

7   Shi L (1994) Primary care, specialty care, and life chances. *International Journal of Health Services.* **24**: 431–58.

8   Shi L, Starfield B, Kennedy BP *et al.* (1999) Income inequality, primary care, and health indicators. *Journal of Family Practice.* **48**: 275–84.

9   Saver B (2002) Financing and organization findings brief. *Academy for Research and Health Care Policy.* **5**: 1–2.

10 Politzer RM, Yoon J, Shi L *et al.* (2001) Inequality in America: the contribution of health centers in reducing and eliminating disparities in access to care. *Medical Care Research and Review.* **58**: 234–48.

11 Gadomski A, Jenkins P and Nichols M (1998) Impact of a Medicaid primary care provider and preventive care on pediatric hospitalization. *Pediatrics.* **101**: E1. http://www.pediatrics.org/cgi/content/full/101/3/e1.

12 Greenfield S, Nelson EC, Zubkoff M *et al.* (1992) Variations in resource utilization among medical specialties and systems of care. Results from the medical outcomes study. *Journal of the American Medical Association.* **267**: 1624–30.

13 Bertakis KD, Callahan EJ, Helms LJ *et al.* (1998) Physician practice styles and patient outcomes: differences between family practice and general internal medicine. *Medical Care.* **36**: 879–91.

14 Bindman AB, Grumbach K, Osmond D *et al.* (1996) Primary care and receipt of preventive services. *Journal of General Internal Medicine.* **11**: 269–76.

15 Hirth RA, Fendrick AM and Chernew ME (1996) Specialist and generalist physicians' adoption of antibiotic therapy to eradicate *Helicobacter pylori* infection. *Medical Care.* **34**: 1199–204.

16 Bartter T and Pratter MR (1996) Asthma: better outcome at lower cost? The role of the expert in the care system. *Chest.* **110**: 1589–96.

17 Harrold LR, Field TS and Gurwitz JH (1999) Knowledge, patterns of care, and outcomes of care for generalists and specialists. *Journal of General Internal Medicine.* **14**: 499–511.

18 Donohoe MT (1998) Comparing generalist and specialty care: discrepancies, deficiencies, and excesses. *Archives of Internal Medicine.* **158**: 1596–608.

19 Grumbach K, Selby JV, Schmittdiel JA *et al.* (1999) Quality of primary care practice in a large HMO according to physician specialty. *Health Services Research.* **34**: 485–502.

20 Starfield B, Lemke KW, Bernhardt T *et al.* (2003) Co-morbidity: implications for the importance of primary care in 'case' management. *Annals of Family Medicine.* **1**: 8–14.

21 Shea S, Misra D, Ehrlich MH *et al.* (1992) Predisposing factors for severe, uncontrolled hypertension in an inner-city minority population. *New England Journal of Medicine.* **327**: 776–81.

22 Parnell SJ, Zalin AM and Clarke CW (1993) Care of diabetic patients in hospital clinics and general practice clinics: a study in Dudley. *British Journal of General Practice.* **43**: 65–9. Erratum: 1993; **43**: 163.

23 Griffin S and Kinmonth A (1998) *Diabetes Care: the effectiveness of systems for routine surveillance for people with diabetes.* Cochrane Library.

24 Kaag ME, Wijkel D and de Jong D (1996) Primary health care replacing hospital care: the effect on quality of care. *International Journal for Quality in Health Care.* **8**: 367–73.

25 Parchman ML and Culler S (1994) Primary care physicians and avoidable hospitalizations. *Journal of Family Practice.* **39**: 123–8.

26 Perrin JM, Greenspan P, Bloom SR *et al.* (1996) Primary care involvement among hospitalized children. *Archives of Pediatrics and Adolescent Medicine.* **150**: 479–86.

27 Ryan S, Riley A, Kang M *et al.* (2001) The effects of regular source of care and health need on medical care use among rural adolescents. *Archives of Pediatrics and Adolescent Medicine.* **155**: 184–90.

28 Jarman B, Gault S, Alves B *et al.* (1999) Explaining differences in English hospital death rates using routinely collected data. *BMJ.* **318**: 1515–20.

29 Gulliford M (2002) Availability of primary care doctors and population health in England: is there an association? *Journal of Public Health Medicine.* **24**: 252–4.

30 Welch WP, Miller ME, Welch HG *et al.* (1993) Geographic variation in expenditures for physicians' services in the United States. *New England Journal of Medicine.* **328**: 621–7.

31 Mark DH, Gottlieb MS, Zellner BB *et al.* (1996) Medicare costs in urban areas and the supply of primary care physicians. *Journal of Family Practice.* **43**: 33–9.

32 Franks P and Fiscella K (1998) Primary care physicians and specialists as personal physicians. Health care expenditures and mortality experience. *Journal of Family Practice.* **47**: 105–9.

33 Starfield B and Shi L (2002) Policy-relevant determinants of health: an international perspective. *Health Policy.* **60**: 201–18.

34 Whittle J, Lin CJ, Lave JR *et al.* (1998) Relationship of provider characteristics to outcomes, process, and costs of care for community-acquired pneumonia. *Medical Care.* **36**: 977–87.

35 Rosser WW (1996) Approach to diagnosis by primary care clinicians and specialists: is there a difference? *Journal of Family Practice.* **42**: 139–44.

36 Shi L and Starfield B (2000) Primary care, income inequality, and self-rated health in the United States: a mixed-level analysis. *International Journal of Health Services.* **30**: 541–55.

37 Shi L, Starfield B, Politzer R *et al.* (2002) Primary care, self-rated health, and reduction in social disparities in health. *Health Services Research.* **37**: 529–50.

38 Roos NP (1979) Who should do the surgery? Tonsillectomy-adenoidectomy in one Canadian province. *Inquiry.* **16**: 73–83.

39   Shi L, Macinko J, Starfield B *et al.* (Submitted 2003) Primary care, infant mortality and low birth weight in US states.

40   Roetzheim RG, Pal N, Gonzalez EC *et al.* (1999) The effects of physician supply on the early detection of colorectal cancer. *Journal of Family Practice.* **48**: 850–8.

41   Shi L (1992) The relationship between primary care and life chances. *Journal of Health Care for the Poor and Underserved.* **3**: 321–35.

42   Farmer FL, Stokes CS, Fiser RH *et al.* (1991) Poverty, primary care and age-specific mortality. *Journal of Rural Health.* **7**: 153–69.

43   Shi L, Starfield B, Politzer R *et al.* (Submitted 2003) Primary care physicians and mortality in the US.

44   Villalbi JR, Guarga A, Pasarin MI *et al.* (1999) An evaluation of the impact of primary care reform on health. *Atencion Primaria.* **24**: 468–74.

45   Shi L, Macinko J and Starfield B (Submitted 2003) Primary care, income inequality and stroke mortality in US states: a longitudinal analysis, 1985–1995.

46   Mansfield CJ, Wilson JL, Kobrinski EJ *et al.* (1999) Premature mortality in the United States: the roles of geographic area, socio-economic status, household type, and availability of medical care. *American Journal of Public Health.* **89**: 893–8.

47   Shi L and Starfield B (2001) The effect of primary care physician supply and income inequality on mortality among blacks and whites in US metropolitan areas. *American Journal of Public Health.* **91**: 1246–50.

48   Castro-Leal F, Dayton J, Demery L *et al.* (2000) Public spending on health care in Africa: do the poor benefit? *Bulletin of the World Health Organization.* **78**: 66–74.

49   Gwatkin DR (2001) The need for equity-oriented health sector reforms. *International Journal of Epidemiology.* **30**: 720–3.

50   Leggetter S, Chaturvedi N, Fuller JH *et al.* (2002) Ethnicity and risk of diabetes-related lower extremity amputation: a population-based, case-control study of African Caribbeans and Europeans in the United Kingdom. *Archives of Internal Medicine.* **162**: 73–8.

51   Starfield B (1991) Primary care and health. A cross-national comparison. *Journal of the American Medical Association.* **266**: 2268–71.

52   Starfield B (1994) Is primary care essential? *Lancet.* **344**: 1129–33.

53   Or Z (2001) Labour Market and Social Policy. Occasional Paper No. 46. *Exploring the Effects of Health Care on Mortality Across OECD Countries.* OECD, Paris.

54   Macinko JA, Starfield B and Shi L (2003) The contribution of primary care systems to health outcomes within Organization for Economic Cooperation and Development (OECD) countries, 1970–1998. *Health Service Research.* **38** (3): 831–65.

55   Starfield B (2001) New paradigms for quality in primary care. *British Journal of General Practice.* **51**: 303–9.

56   van den Akker M, Buntinx F, Metsemakers JF *et al.* (1998) Multimorbidity in general practice: prevalence, incidence, and determinants of co-occurring chronic and recurrent diseases. *Journal of Clinical Epidemiology.* **51**: 367–75.

57 Lamberts H, Wood M and Hofmans-Okkes I (1993) *The International Classification of Primary Care in the European Community*. Oxford University Press, Oxford/New York.

58 Feachem RG, Sekhri NK and White KL (2002) Getting more for their dollar: a comparison of the NHS with California's Kaiser Permanente. *BMJ*. **324**: 135–41.

CHAPTER 3

Quality and standards in general practice

Richard Baker

Introduction

General practitioners in the UK have discussed quality and standards since the creation of the NHS in 1948. A possible explanation for this preoccupation is that quality and standards have been poor and efforts to improve unsuccessful. An alternative explanation is that quality and standards have been acceptable, but GPs have wished to achieve even more. The conclusion of this chapter is that the truth lies between these extremes: GPs have been ambitious in their goals for quality and standards, but they have not always achieved as much as they hoped. This is partly explained by variation in performance between practitioners, but also by the resources available and the organisation and leadership of health services.

This chapter first discusses the definition of quality, concentrating on one that takes account of the judgements of professionals, patients and policy makers in the context of the legal and social codes that govern healthcare. The methods of quality assessment are then considered, and it is suggested that in future an increased emphasis will be placed on outcomes. In the next section, the level of quality and success in its improvement are discussed, concluding with a personal view of the key elements required for quality improvement. The final section asks whether GPs can justifiably celebrate their achievements in quality and standards.

What is quality in general practice?

There are several definitions of quality, although none is entirely satisfactory. Most definitions are lists of attributes of care that can be regarded as more or less desirable. The most familiar example is that proposed by Maxwell (*see* Box 3.1).[1] In an alternative definition, care was divided into care for individuals

> **Box 3.1** Dimensions of healthcare quality
>
> - Access to services
> - Relevance to need (for the whole community)
> - Effectiveness (for individual patients)
> - Equity (fairness)
> - Social acceptability

(access, clinical effectiveness, interpersonal effectiveness) and care for populations (consisting of care for individuals plus equity and efficiency).[2] Quality of care in general practice has been defined as being better when more rather than less attention is given to physical and psychological co-morbidity at consultations, when more health promotion is provided, less medication prescribed and patients express more satisfaction.[3] In seeking to describe the core nature of their work, leading thinkers in each generation of GPs have written on the features of good general practice. The work of Toon is a recent example of this tradition that has played a key role in the development of general practice in the last 50 years, and presents a very different perspective on quality to that encapsulated in Maxwell's tidy list.[4]

Many will be familiar with Donabedian's most widely used suggestion, namely that quality of care may be classified into structure, process or outcome elements.[5] However, this is only a short extract from a complex discussion from which several definitions emerge, including for example that quality is the extent to which the benefits of care exceed the harms. In recognition of the multiplicity of definitions of quality, a post-modern or developmental approach has been suggested, in which the existence of different perspectives is accepted.[6] Attempts to produce a unified definition and associated set of indicators are avoided, indicators being developed locally by those who will be judged by them.

Another of Donabedian's definitions, described as the unifying model, anticipates and largely addresses many of these difficulties. In this definition, quality of care is a property of, and a judgement upon, an element of care. The judges may be categorised as patients, professionals or managers of care, and each group uses a different perspective when judging quality. Furthermore, individuals will also have their own particular perspectives. And judgement, of course, involves more than merely measurement, it relies also on the values, expectations, beliefs, prejudices and preferences of the individuals and groups judging care. Most of the other definitions assume that quality is a property of care only, and if it can be specified sufficiently clearly, it can be readily measured and monitored as improvement is attempted. But the idea of judgement makes clear that quality is much more complex.[7]

In Figure 3.1, Donabedian's original idea is presented as a model of quality in healthcare. The three groups of judges of quality are patients (to include all present and potential users of healthcare services), professionals (all those providing care, including doctors and nurses) and planners (to include managers and policy makers in government or insurers in those countries in which care is funded in this way). Inevitably there will be some agreement between the three parties on what constitutes quality, but there will also be some disagreement. It might be argued that the most desirable situation would be complete agreement between patients, professionals and planners. They would then be likely to work together to achieve their shared aim. In some countries, there may be a reasonable consensus and the goals of health service policy will not then be controversial. However, in the UK, this has not been the case for at least the last 20 years.

The extent of disagreement will vary from time to time, and in consequence a mechanism is required to bring about an amicable balance. That mechanism consists of the written and unwritten codes that govern healthcare. Some of these codes are contained in legislation, others in health service regulations, and others are implicit but accepted social conventions or ethical principles, or even merely habits.[8] For example, a patient's demand for penicillin for a viral throat infection can be refused by a GP because both health service regulations and legal codes give the practitioner authority to make this decision. In this

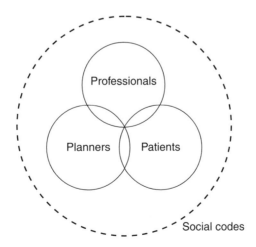

Figure 3.1   A model of quality in healthcare.

case, it is the professional's view of quality that prevails. On the other hand, a patient with advanced cancer advised by the doctor to try a highly toxic treatment can choose to ignore the advice, an example in which the patient's view of quality takes precedence. At the group level, planners and professionals may determine that a treatment such as beta-interferon is not cost-effective, but patient organisations may come to a different conclusion. In this case, legislation favours the planners.

The model of quality also highlights the potential consequences of a major breach of the codes by the profession. The most obvious recent example is retention of body parts following post-mortem at Alder Hey hospital.[9] It subsequently emerged that this practice was widespread and that the consent of relatives had been largely taken for granted. When planners and patients discover that doctors have unwittingly or deliberately ignored the codes, trust in the profession is impaired and a review of regulations inevitably follows. Such events have not been common in the last 50 years of general practice, but there have been several recently, some of which have involved GPs. Consequently, we find ourselves in a period in which the codes that govern the practice of medicine are being revised and extended.

In the decades before the recent upheaval, a continuing debate began among GPs on whether they should resist planners' and patients' perspectives on quality or whether they should acknowledge the progressive development of these new views, and react by introducing professional reforms. The stance of the Royal College of General Practitioners (RCGP) has generally been on the side of the modernisers, as this quotation from a policy statement in 1985 illustrates:[10]

> We live in a time when powerful forces are creating unprecedented change in our approach to health and illness. ... The Statement confirms our confidence in the capacity and will of general practice to adapt and modernize, so to fulfil its growing clinical commitments to patients whilst retaining the central characteristic of personal care which people clearly want and appreciate.

The College was created by GPs who were aware that the expectations of policy makers and patients were gradually changing, and it has since served as a focus for discussion on the profession's response. The report of the steering committee that launched the then College of General Practitioners on 19 November 1952 makes explicit the aspiration of the College's founders to develop a higher standard of general practice.[11] GPs' relationships with patients in the community make them aware of the views people hold about health services, but doctors who work in hospitals are relatively insulated from such views. Consequently, GPs have a special role to play on behalf of all doctors in being sensitive to changes in the implicit codes that govern the choice between different perspectives on quality.

General practitioners' own ideas on what constitutes quality are always developing, and there is a continuing debate on what is important. From one perspective, the relationship between patient and doctor is the key, as exemplified in the writings of Michael Balint, a psychoanalyst whose work in the 1950s/1960s helped GPs understand the psychology of the doctor–patient relationship. His best-known work is probably *The Doctor, His Patient and the Illness*, published in 1957. A broader perspective can be found in the patient-centred clinical method, founded on the principle that the GP is committed to the person rather than to a particular body of knowledge or group of diseases.[12] The GP has been argued to have the key roles of interpreter at the interface between illness and disease, and of witness to the patient's experience.[13] A rather different view can be found in the argument for evidence-based practice which asserts that there is a gap between best research evidence and doctors' daily clinical practice.[14] The solution is the development of skills and policies for using research evidence with patients, and perhaps also methods for substituting the autonomy of clinicians with clinical practice guided by electronic decision support systems. The concept of the personal doctor is also under challenge. The growth of primary healthcare teams and the creation of primary care organisations reflect a view that the relationship between the patient and the health service is equally if not more important than the relationship between the patient and the individual GP.[15]

The different views on what is quality general practice have been blended in a recent report of the RCGP and the General Practitioners Committee of the British Medical Association (BMA). *Good Medical Practice for General Practitioners* sets out the standards expected of GPs as a foundation for the introduction of revalidation.[16] The 18 aspects of care addressed together with example criteria that describe the excellent and unacceptable GP are shown in Table 3.1. It should be noted that the standards apply to individual GPs and not general practices or primary healthcare teams. Nevertheless, they represent the most complete current amalgamation of the different perspectives on quality in general practice. Clinical competence, evidence-based practice, commitment to the individual and the needs of the population, and responsibility for working with others are all included. *Good Medical Practice for General Practitioners* is therefore a significant step in the evolution of the discipline. Not only does it serve as the basis for revalidation, but it is also a statement of values to which all GPs at all stages in their careers can aspire.

Assessment of quality

During the last 50 years, three stages in the development of quality assessment methods can be distinguished, and these may be roughly grouped into structure, process and outcome phases (Table 3.2). In the first phase, the aim was to ensure that the doctor was adequately educated. Initially, emphasis was placed on the demonstration of worthiness through experience of practice and seniority.

Table 3.1 The aspects of care addressed in *Good Medical Practice for General Practitioners*,[16] September 2002, with selected examples of criteria describing the excellent and the unacceptable GP*

Aspect of practice	Example criteria	
	The excellent GP	*The unacceptable GP*
Clinical care	Maintains knowledge and skills, and is aware of limits of competence	Consistently ignores, interrupts or contradicts patients
	Considers relevant psychological and social factors as well as physical ones	Fails to elicit important parts of the history
	Is selective but systematic when examining patients	Gives treatments that are inconsistent with best practice or evidence
Keeping records	Records appropriate information for all contacts	Keeps records which are incomplete or illegible, and contain inaccurate details or gratuitously derogatory remarks
	Respects patient's right to confidentiality	Consistently consults without records
Access and availability	An effective system for responding to emergencies	Provides no opportunity for patients to talk to a doctor or nurse on the phone
	Opening hours that meet the needs of the patient population	Has no knowledge of the qualifications of locums employed in the practice or ignores doubts about their ability
Emergencies	Reviews the care of emergency cases as part of clinical meetings	Does not maintain resuscitation skills
Effective use of resources	Takes resources into account when choosing between treatments of similar effectiveness	Consistently prescribes unnecessary or ineffective treatments
Keeping up to date	Up to date with developments in clinical practice and regularly reviews knowledge and performance	Is hostile to external audit or advice
	Uses a range of methods to monitor different aspects of care and to meet educational needs	Has little insight into their knowledge or performance

Continued

Table 3.1   Continued

Aspect of practice	Example criteria	
	The excellent GP	*The unacceptable GP*
Information about your services	Leaves clear messages if an answerphone is used	Does not have a practice leaflet, or has one which is untrue or self-promoting
Maintaining trust	Involves patients in decisions about their care Respects the right of patients to refuse treatments or tests	Exploits relationships with patients to their own advantage Fails to obtain patients' consent to treatment
Avoiding discrimination and prejudice	Is aware of how their personal beliefs could affect the care offered to the patient, and takes care not to impose their own beliefs and values	Provides better care to some patients than others as a result of their own prejudices
If things go wrong	Apologises for themselves or for the practice staff Cooperates with any investigation arising from a complaint	Does not acknowledge or attempt to rectify any mistakes that occur Allows a complaint to influence their care of the patient adversely
Working with colleagues and in teams	Understands the health needs of the local population and tries to ensure that the primary healthcare team has the skills to meet those needs Aims to develop an organisation which offers personal and professional development opportunities to its staff	Does not attempt to meet members of the primary care team (e.g. district nurses or health visitors), or even know who they are Delegates tasks to other members of the team for which they do not have the appropriate skills
Referring patients	Makes appropriate judgements about patients who need referral Accompanies referrals with the information needed by the specialist to make an efficient evaluation of the patient's problem	Does not refer patients when specialist care is necessary Consistently dismisses patients' requests for a second opinion

Continued

Table 3.1 Continued

Aspect of practice	Example criteria	
	The excellent GP	*The unacceptable GP*
Accepting posts	Provides the care that they have agreed to provide	Holds no personal responsibility for care that he or she has agreed to provide
Teaching, training, appraisal and assessment	The excellent teacher has personal commitment to teaching and learning Shows a willingness to develop both themselves and other doctors or students, through education, audit and peer review	Fails to take appropriate action when the performance of a learner is inadequate Puts patients at risk by allowing the learner to practise beyond the limits of their competence
Research	Protects patients' rights, and makes sure that they are not disadvantaged by taking part in research	Provides inaccurate or false data
Financial and commercial dealings	Is an example of financial probity in society	Seeks personal financial gain from their patients other than the normal remuneration expected from their job
Providing references	Is honest and objective in comments made in references, and does not miss out important information	Includes comments in references (favourable or unfavourable) which are based largely on personal prejudice
Health and performance	Is aware when a colleague's performance, conduct or health might be putting patients at risk Realises when their own performance is unsafe, e.g. through illness	Takes no advice, nor offers any to the colleague concerned Denies or actively conceals their own ill health

*For full details, see http://www.rcgp.org.uk/rcgp/corporate/position/good_med_prac/gmp06.pdf

In 1965, an examination for entry to the College was introduced (five candidates sat the first examination and all passed), and it has since progressively become both more popular and also more complex. The culmination of the structure phase came with the introduction in 1980 of mandatory vocational training before approval to begin independent practice.

Table 3.2 Stages in the development of quality assessment in general practice

Stages	Measures used for assessment of quality
1 Structure	Length of time as a GP Participation in professional activities Demonstration of fitness for independent practice through completion of vocational training Demonstration of knowledge through an examination
2 Process	Immunisation rate targets Audits of care of selected conditions Objective measures of personal performance such as Membership or Fellowship by Assessment
3 Outcome	Patient satisfaction Symptom questionnaires Intermediate outcomes Mortality

The structure phase was based on the belief that if it had been established that the new doctor had the necessary knowledge and skills, subsequent performance would be of acceptable quality. This belief was of course incomplete, and attention moved from ensuring that the structure (the doctor) was competent on entry to the profession to determining whether performance was adequate when in practice. The process phase of quality assessment included growth in interest in clinical audit during the 1980s, and its formal support by local groups from 1991. Assessment of aspects of the process of care was introduced into the 1990 contract for GPs, and the recently announced replacement of that contract will include the collection of detailed data about the care of people with selected chronic illnesses. Although improvement in practice information systems makes use of large quantities of data possible, it does not ensure the validity of recorded data nor the informed interpretation of the findings. Furthermore, the approach does not reflect the range of values encapsulated in *Good Medical Practice for General Practitioners*.[16]

General practitioners have addressed some of these problems by themselves developing methods for the assessment of process. The College has programmes for Membership and Fellowship by Assessment for individual practitioners, an initiative to help primary care organisations develop the performance of teams (Quality Team Development) and a procedure undertaken by practices to recognise high standards (the Quality Practice Award). The General Practitioners Committee of the BMA has produced a primary care organisation assessment that includes a range of performance indicators, and projects to support the creation of a partnership between doctors and patients.

Nevertheless, some aspects of care are impossible to quantify. Qualitative assessment methods can be used in research studies to accommodate this problem, but they are difficult to use routinely. Outcome assessment may offer some solutions to these difficulties, and the start of an outcome phase to quality assessment in general practice is now perceptible. The most obvious example is the fashion for patient surveys. Patients' views about or satisfaction with the care they have received is an outcome of care, and the collection of information from samples of patients using standard questionnaires is relatively convenient. A national survey of patient opinion has been undertaken in England, and patients' dissatisfaction with access to primary care was a key finding.[17] Many practices have undertaken surveys in recent years, and primary care organisations are following suit.

Surveys have limitations. They provide us with answers from large numbers of people to the questions we put to them. They do not, however, help us understand which questions are really important. Detailed interviews of small numbers of patients can go some way to addressing this problem, but the method requires expertise and can be costly. Even though we learn to understand our patients during consultations, we have not yet found a reliable way to translate that understanding into methods for designing practice policies and service routines that meet their particular preferences.

The collection of data about clinical outcomes in general practice is also difficult. The numbers of patients in a general practice with a particular condition are small, outcome is influenced by many factors other than prior treatment, and can be delayed long after treatment is given. Health symptom questionnaires may sometimes be helpful, for example in estimating the severity of symptoms in asthma, angina or depression, but they require time and expertise to administer and analyse. Intermediate outcomes are the most promising measures for immediate use, including, for example, blood pressure, cholesterol and glucose control. The disadvantage of these measures is that adequate control can sometimes be difficult or impossible to achieve without the creation of intolerable side effects. Despite these reservations, however, assessment of outcome should not be dismissed as impossible or irrelevant. New measures are being developed, and new techniques are available for the statistical analysis of outcomes involving small numbers of patients. It is probable, therefore, that within a short period, practical measures of outcome for use in general practice will be available.

Quality improvement

If after reading Collings' damning report on general practice published in 1950,[18] you were, today, to walk into virtually any general practice in Britain, you would need no convincing that dramatic improvements in quality have taken place. The modern practice, with its primary healthcare team, clinical equipment, computer information systems and special clinics is very different from the practice run by the isolated practitioner from a room in the family home 52 years ago.

It is not surprising, however, that there has been much change over such a long period; the question is whether there has been sufficient change. The challenge facing general practice is not limited to keeping pace with historical trends, but also to responding to the evolving expectations of the public, the discovery of new or re-evaluation of established forms of clinical management and the needs of different communities. How successful have we been in relation to these three aspects of practice?

Expectations

There is little evidence about the extent to which we have responded to the expectations of the public and it is important not to allow our personal or professional perspectives to cloud the assessment. General practice has been a leading advocate among the medical disciplines for patient-centred care, and the GP is the personal doctor who blends science with art to best serve the unique needs of each individual patient. This tradition has been the driving force behind the creation of postgraduate training programmes and has led to the introduction of the teaching of consultation skills in undergraduate medical schools. There is, then, much to celebrate.

A slightly different picture emerges when the issue of access to GPs is considered, as the 1998 national survey of patient opinion has demonstrated.[17] Of the 100 000 people sent questionnaires, 65% responded, of whom 81% had consulted a GP in the past 12 months. In general, people were content with general practice and GPs. However, access was heavily criticised, with one in four respondents who had consulted a GP having to wait more than four days to see the doctor of their choice, and 5% having to wait eight days or longer. Concern about access has prompted new approaches in practices that include telephone triage and nurse consultations, but has also led to the creation of alternative sources of primary care, including walk-in centres and the telephone service NHS Direct. Unsatisfactory access is one consequence of prolonged under-investment in general practice, and GPs cannot be held totally responsible, but the access problem serves to illustrate the consequences of failing to respond to the expectations of the public. Perhaps we should have identified this problem before the national survey and done more to alleviate it, rather than waiting for the introduction of national policy developments that are potentially detrimental to personal primary care.

Clinical management

How effectively has general practice responded to new therapies or techniques, or new evidence about established therapies? There are examples of important and relatively rapid responses to such evidence. For example, the switch to modern anti-hypertensives in place of methyl dopa or reserpine, the decline in the use of barbiturates, the introduction of clinics for people with diabetes or the wide use of statins all took place relatively quickly. However, there are reasons for believing that care in general practice is not always in accordance with best current evidence. In a systematic review of 90 studies of care in general practice, 80 of which were undertaken in the UK, Seddon and colleagues[19] found that in almost all studies the processes of care did not attain the standards set out in national guidelines or set by the researchers themselves. The potential explanations include unrealistic standards, patients' preferences being at variance with the evidence and resources being insufficient to provide adequate time or staff. However, findings from studies showing that no practice had managed to check the fundi of more than 49% of people with diabetes, or had prescribed beta-blockers to more than 47% of eligible patients after myocardial infarction should give rise to concern. Wide variations in performance between practices is usually observed in quality assessment studies, and a proportion of this variation cannot be explained by clinical factors, patient preference or matters outside the control of the GP. It must be concluded that the effectiveness of aspects of care in at least some practices could be improved, and the last decade of initiatives that include clinical audit, clinical governance, national guidelines and incentive payments is evidence that this conclusion has been shared by policy makers.

Needs of different communities

One explanation for variation between practices is that different patient communities have different needs. Through close contact with their communities and their understanding of patients, GPs are well placed to tailor their services to the needs of local communities. They can also act as advocates for their patients in the development of health policies and decisions about the use of resources. There are outstanding examples of GPs who have successfully fulfilled the dual role of providing tailored services and advocacy on behalf of deprived communities, yet there is also evidence that the inverse care law is still active. The care of people with diabetes offers one example. There is evidence to suggest that general practices in more deprived areas have been slower to take up additional payments for structured diabetes care, with practice characteristics being associated with the likelihood of diabetes reviews in deprived areas.[20] In another study, patients of practices in more deprived areas were found to be less likely to have routine examinations and checks of glycated haemoglobin.[21]

Improving quality

It is reasonable to conclude that general practice has devoted considerable effort to responding to the evolving expectations of the public, the discovery of new treatments and the needs of different communities, and has been rewarded by some successes. Nevertheless, a great deal remains to be done. Although the poor performance of a very few GPs may explain some of the disappointing progress, much has also depended on factors extraneous to the practice, including in particular resources, policies and health service management. Policy reform has now become routine, but until recently most quality improvement activities were targeted at the health professional.

There is now a growing body of research evidence about the impact of different methods of implementing change in performance. The interventions studied include guidelines, feedback, educational outreach, reminders and delegation within teams. GPs have not been slow to use these methods. However, since these have been discovered to be of variable effectiveness at best, other approaches have been introduced in the absence of detailed evaluation, for example continuous quality improvement or system re-engineering. More recently, the difficulties of quality improvement have been explained by the idea of complexity. Healthcare organisations are complex adaptive systems and it is inappropriate to seek an ideal quality improvement plan. The aim should be a 'good enough plan' that is put into operation, observed and modified in the light of experience.

There are many systematic reviews of the evidence about the effectiveness of different implementation strategies, and these reviews have been summarised in other publications.[22,23] Instead of repeating these summaries, I offer a conclusion based on personal experience rather than experimental evidence. The following ingredients appear to me to be important for quality and for improving quality:

- skilled and motivated health professionals
- functional teams that can work together to set priorities, agree and implement practical plans, and evaluate their progress
- organisations that see the support and development of individuals and teams as the first priority in achieving the levels of quality expected by patients
- leaders who first listen in order to develop an understanding of the organisation, its people and circumstances, and who then create a clear and constant purpose, and generate an organisational culture and structure that enables individuals and teams to work to achieve that purpose.

Of course, time, money and sufficient numbers of staff all help, and a minimum level of all three is essential, but they do not compensate for a deficiency in these four ingredients.

Conclusions

Should general practice feel entitled to celebrate its record in relation to quality and standards? On the basis of the discussion in this chapter, the answer to this question cannot be an unqualified 'Yes'. *Good Medical Practice For General Practitioners*[16] provides a reasonable basis for defining quality and serving as the foundation for standards, although it would be wrong to claim that GPs unanimously agree that it includes everything of importance.

We are rather uncertain about what aspects of care should be addressed, and the latest contract for GPs has opted for assessing a long list of process measures. A more balanced approach would include assessment of consultation competence,[24] outcomes and partnerships with patients.

As far as quality improvement is concerned, we have expended considerable effort, with some success. However, wide variations in performance can still be found, and some groups of patients remain particularly poorly served.

However, this downbeat conclusion is only part of the picture. The restrictions placed on general practice must bear much of the responsibility for limiting progress in quality and standards. Whilst the past 20 years of NHS policy have seen many changes and increases in investment, the needs of general practice have been regularly overlooked. Reforms have been designed to address the difficulties facing secondary care, and the new resources have almost always been swallowed up by the needs of hospitals. If general practice is recognised as having been an afterthought in policy terms, then its achievements have been commendable. Despite relative neglect, much has been achieved. We should in particular celebrate the work of numerous individual practitioners who have struggled to bring about improvements, and who in many instances have transformed aspects of care and the quality of life of their patients. We need to address the remaining pockets of poor performance, but there is no escape from the conclusion that general practice has done as well as, if not a little better than, it has been allowed to by the constraints under which it has operated. By and large, therefore, we should celebrate the individuals who have delivered general practice, but regret the circumstances in which they have had to work.

References

1   Maxwell RJ (1984) Quality assessment in health. *BMJ.* **288**: 1470–2.

2   Campbell SM, Roland MO and Buetow S (2000) Defining quality of care. *Social Science and Medicine.* **51**: 1611–25.

3   Howie JGR, Heaney D and Maxwell M (1997) *Measuring Quality in General Practice.* Occasional paper 75. Royal College of General Practitioners, London.

4   Toon P (1999) *Towards a Philosophy of General Practice: a study of the virtuous practitioner*. Occasional Paper 78. Royal College of General Practitioners, London.

5   Donabedian A (1980) *Explorations in Quality Assessment and Monitoring. Volume 1: the definition of quality and approaches to its assessment*. Health Administration Press, Ann Arbor.

6   Greenhalgh T and Eversley J (1999) *Quality in General Practice*. King's Fund, London.

7   Baker R (1988) *Practice Assessment and Quality Care*. Occasional Paper 39. Royal College of General Practitioners, London.

8   Baker R (2001) Principles of quality improvement. Part one – defining quality. *Journal of Clinical Governance*. **9**: 89–91.

9   Royal Liverpool Children's Inquiry Report (2001) House of Commons, London.

10   Royal College of General Practitioners (1985) *Quality in General Practice*. Policy statement 2. Royal College of General Practitioners, London.

11   Barber GO, Hunt JH and Rogers TA (1983) The work of the steering committee, and the birth of the College. In: Fry J, Lord Hunt of Fawley and Pinsent RJFH (eds) *A History of the Royal College of General Practitioners*. MTP Press Ltd, Lancaster.

12   McWhinney IR (1997) *A Textbook of Family Medicine* (2e). Oxford University Press, Oxford.

13   Heath I (1995) *The Mystery of General Practice*. Nuffield Provincial Hospitals Trust, London.

14   Silagy C and Weller D (1998) Evidence-based practice in primary care: an introduction. In: Silagy C and Haines A (eds) *Evidence-based Practice in Primary Care*. BMJ Books, London.

15   Wilke G and Freeman S (2001) *How to be a Good Enough GP*. Radcliffe Medical Press, Oxford.

16   Royal College of General Practitioners and General Practitioners Committee (2002) *Good Medical Practice for General Practitioners*. Royal College of General Practitioners, London.

17   Airey C, Bruster S, Erens B *et al.* (1999) *National Survey of NHS Patients. General Practice 1998*. NHS Executive, London. http://193.32.28.83/public/nhssurvey.htm.

18   Collings J (1950) General practice in England today: a reconnaissance. *Lancet*. **1**: 555–85.

19   Seddon ME, Marshall MN, Campbell SM *et al.* (2001) Systematic review of studies of quality of clinical care in general practice in the UK, Australia and New Zealand. *Quality in Health Care*. **10**: 152–8.

20   Goyder EC, McNally PG and Botha JL (2000) Inequalities in access to diabetes care: evidence from a historical cohort study. *Quality in Health Care*. **9**: 85–9.

21   Khunti K, Ganguli S, Baker R *et al.* (2001) Features of primary care associated with variations in process and outcome of care of people with diabetes. *British Journal of General Practice*. **51**: 356–60.

22 NHS Centre for Reviews and Dissemination (1999) Getting evidence into practice. *Effective Health Care.* **5** (1): 1–16.

23 Baker R, Stevenson K, Shaw E *et al.* (2002) Review of the evidence. In: National Institute for Clinical Excellence *Principles for Best Practice in Clinical Audit.* Radcliffe Medical Press, Oxford.

24 McKinley RK, Fraser RC and Baker R (2001) Suggested model for directly assessing and enhancing clinical competence and performance in clinician revalidation. *BMJ.* **322**: 712–15.

CHAPTER 4

Celebrating European cooperation in general practice

Chris van Weel

It was shortly after I had joined the rank and file of general practice that I was invited to attend a meeting of the Rotterdam faculty of the Dutch College of GPs – the biannual exchange with the then Teesside faculty of the RCGP. Waiting with the others for our British guests provided the opportunity of a swift introduction to the Rotterdam general practice network and there I was introduced, among others, to Professor Heert Dokter, who would later become my supervisor for my MD thesis. Thirty years later the academic programme is still fresh in my mind: for the first time I witnessed the reporting of research that resulted from settings comparable to my own practice. Differences between presentations of our own and those of our guests were few and minor. It was implicitly obvious that we shared professional concepts, terminology and values. And where circumstances differed this offered an opportunity for exciting reflections. Non-medicalised home deliveries in the Netherlands triggered a profound discussion on the implications of a natural and holistic approach to healthcare. Home treatment of myocardial infarction – which went against the prevailing Dutch routine – gave insight into the risks and dangers of high technology care.

I soon found out those exchanges with UK general practice were common-place in Dutch general practice. There was also some contact with Scandinavian GPs. However that was about the extent of European cooperation in general practice. We would occasionally bump into colleagues from Belgium and Germany, and though these contacts were enjoyed and appreciated, it seldom led to professional reflection. GPs in these countries worked under such completely different circumstances (*see* Figure 4.1)[1] that it was impossible to recognise their everyday reality. In particular, the Flemish–Dutch exchanges often circled around the conclusion – subscribed to by both parties – that the difference in health-care systems was too great!

In present-day Europe general practice is regarded an essential part of health-care, responsible for medical care in the community, with a special emphasis on

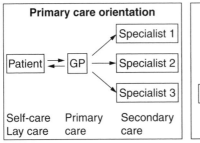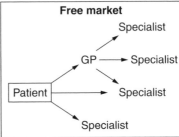

Figure 4.1 Healthcare structure and access to care.[1]

the early diagnosis and treatment of illness, continuity of care and the tailoring of medical interventions to patients' personal circumstances. Its mission is articulated in *The European Definition of General Practice/Family Medicine* as are the competencies practitioners must demonstrate:[2]

- the management of patients, including the interventions made by other specialists
- person-centred care, which requires the ability to establish and develop an effective doctor–patient relationship over time
- problem-solving skills that enable clinical decisions to be made when signs and symptoms are not well established and there is a low probability of major disease
- coping with uncertainty in diagnosis, treatment and prevention without resorting to undue use of investigations and referral
- a comprehensive approach that allows the simultaneous management of different health problems in the individual and combines prevention, health promotion and treatment
- a community orientation in understanding the health needs of the population in which the GP is practising; and a holistic use of the bio-psychosocial model, taking in cultural and existential dimensions.

In this way, GPs in Europe share a responsibility to provide an environment of medical care that is safe for patients and protects them against the negative effects of excessive medical and hospital care. This coming together of European general practice now even includes the teaching of medical undergraduates in general practice: the European Union Socrates programme *Primary Medical Care*[3] provides a framework for exchange between England, Belgium, Germany and the Netherlands, with recent extensions to Sweden and Scotland and hopefully soon Austria, Italy and Slovenia. Whilst learning about the essential orientation of different healthcare systems and the role of general practice, medical students are able to improve their primary care-based clinical skills. What has emerged is that there is sufficient common ground for teaching.

Changes in the structure of healthcare were abundant in Europe during the 1990s, but despite the fact that 'healthcare reform' is a common European issue that is likely to stay with us, the fundamental differences under which GPs work have remained substantial. In the UK, Denmark and the Netherlands, GPs are still responsible for a defined practice population, a characteristic notably absent in most central European countries. Working in competition with other medical providers in the community is the reality in the European continent with the exception of the Iberian peninsula, Scandinavia and the Netherlands. Given the substantial differences in systems and structures that GPs work under throughout Europe, it is intriguing to ask what has brought European-based GPs together in the past two decades?

In my view this is due to a number of developments. The first has to do with the unravelling of the content of general practice. Responsibility for a defined practice population, or constant competition with other medical specialists for the favours of patients, pose completely different perspectives on how to run a practice. Understandably this is what initial comparisons touch upon. But GPs direct their care in response to patients' needs, so, irrespective of health service structure and regulations, patients' health problems form the basis of the care GPs provide. In particular, through the development and field-testing of international disease classifications for general practice have the needs of patients become clear,[4] highlighting the fact that patients by and large seek (primary) medical care for the same health problems even when the system differences yielded differences in management. A case in point was the thesis by Jan De Maeseneer[5] that analysed morbidity in Belgian general practice and described a near similar pattern to Dutch morbidity data. It finally silenced Flemish–Dutch debates over the 'best' system but it opened a whole new area for analysis, for example of practitioner-initiated differences in prescribing, home visits or other 'system-influenced' factors. In other words, European GPs developed a methodology to look 'behind' the facade of system-related data, and this opened the possibility of the *joint* development of the academic content of general practice. This in fact did lead to the issues addressed in *The European Definition of General Practice/Family Medicine*.[2] With hindsight this was old news as back in 1961 Kerr White *et al.* discussed the ecology of medical care[6] as a phenomenon independent of the structure of care (*see* Figure 4.2).

The fall of the Berlin Wall in 1989 recreated civil societies in Central and Eastern Europe and healthcare was a key part of that process. With primary care an integral part of healthcare reform, there was an urgent need to promote, to an outside audience, the strength and virtues of general practice. It was best to work together in international partnerships rather than have internal feuds over 'best systems'. It also provided an excellent opportunity to look behind 'the system' at the core of general practice. The rapid successes achieved in Poland,

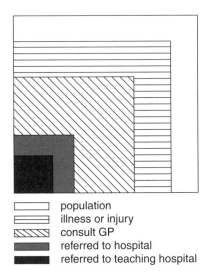

population
illness or injury
consult GP
referred to hospital
referred to teaching hospital

Figure 4.2   Morbidity in the community.[6]

Estonia and Slovenia were of the utmost importance for general practice: they stated in the most unambiguous terms that general practice had a mission to accomplish.

The third development that took place may not look significant, but I believe it was: the change from Societas Internationalis Medicinae Generalis (SIMG) as the binding force of European general practice to World Organisation of National Colleges and Academies of General Practice (WONCA Europe). In 1995 this transfer materialised and it signalled a change-over from a central European, mainly German-speaking organisation to an organisation of academic general practice in the global Anglo-American traditions. With it went the traditions of tri-lingual (German–English–French) simultaneously translated meetings to be replaced by 'English-only' conferences. The initial fear was that this would restrict the involvement of those GPs from central European, German-speaking countries, but the opposite has happened: since the creation of WONCA Europe the level of participation has grown – both in terms of individual practitioners and in the number of national academic general practice organisations. Speaking one common language secured a fundamental principle: meetings were to foster the exchange of professional experience and to enhance the involvement of individuals. What mattered were concepts and ideas, not primarily the language these ideas and concepts were formulated in. With hindsight, simultaneous translation – with the objective to clarify matters – did much to disguise misunderstanding. Forcing European GPs to address each other directly in a common language turned out to be a powerful method to build a common frame of reference.

In summary, European GPs in 2003 find themselves working under healthcare systems as varied and diverse as in the 1950s, when many started to tap into the experience and expertise of the RCGP. What has changed though is the understanding that irrespective of healthcare systems, the generic concepts of general practice remain true. No longer tied by these restrictions, general practice has established itself as an integral part of European healthcare.

With exchange of experience now the rule rather than the exception, it is pertinent to ask who benefits from this. It is obvious that general practice in most of the 'new' countries has benefited greatly: the intensive contacts with the UK and the Netherlands have enabled them to speed up their progress without the most basic serendipity of having to learn entirely from one's own experience. What it has brought to the established organisations is probably more difficult to say. But I think organisations like the RCGP or the Dutch college are likely to share my personal experience highlighted in the introduction of this article: I met my mentor Heert Dokter and established a long working relationship with him. I was also introduced at that meeting in 1974 to Frans Huygen, the doyen of Dutch general practice. Taking part in international meetings may be helpful for others, but it definitely encourages a more profound reflection of one's own situation. So, international cooperation is an opportunity to altruistically put one's own experience at the disposal of others, but it also leads to better self-understanding, and that is where the next phase of future professional development usually starts.

References

1   van Weel C (1999) The international perspective of general practice research. *European Journal of General Practice.* **5**: 110–15.

2   WONCA Europe (2000) *The European Definition of General Practice/Family Medicine.* WONCA Europe.

3   van Weel C (1999) The European Union Socrates programme: *Primary Medical Care – A Five-year Review.* University of Nijmegen, Nijmegen.

4   Lamberts H, Meads S and Wood M (1984) Waarom gaat iemand naar de huisarts? Een internationale studie met de Reason for Encounter Classification. [Why go to a doctor? An international study with the Reason for Encounter Classification – synopsis in English.] *Huisarts en Wetenschap.* **27**: 234–44.

5   De Maeseneer J (1989) Huisartsgeneeskunde: een verkenning. Dissertation (English summary). University of Ghent, Belgium.

6   White KL, Williams TF and Greenberg BC (1961) The ecology of medical care. *New England Journal of Medicine.* **265**: 885–992.

CHAPTER 5

The value of general practice to the NHS

Mike Pringle

Introduction

In times of change professional groups naturally fear for their future. The National Health Service seems to have been in constant turmoil since 1989,[1] and general practitioners worry that society, the NHS or other health professionals will value and reward them less, that their future will be marginalised.

While the role of general practice changes insidiously year by year, it is during major reforms that our awareness of shifts in roles and responsibilities is heightened. Since the publication of *The NHS Plan*[2] for England in the summer of 2000 we have seen a range of proposals to change the roles of health professionals,[3,4] change the GP contract,[5] increase accountability[6] and tighten performance management.[7]

The fact that primary care is moving to the centre of the NHS, taking responsibility for commissioning appropriate services from all sectors using nearly three-quarters of all state health funding, might be seen to confirm the view from abroad that general practice is a jewel in Britain's health crown.[8] Many of us believe that general practice offers an effective, efficient service that is highly valued by patients.

In times such as these we need to make the case for general practice explicitly. Inevitably the case will be presented to politicians and the public using pragmatic arguments and relative assessments. However, we cannot make that case effectively if we do not believe in a set of shared values that underpin our confidence. Without those values we are liable to the charge of professional protectionism; with them we are defending the interests of the public and patients.

So, this chapter looks at our care values. Some might regard this as an exercise in pedantry – our values are implicit and well understood. Others might feel that debates on our values dominated the development of our discipline[9] and that the case has been made. For many, however, including myself, our values need reviewing and restating because the world in which we live and work is changing around us. In this context, our values remain steady but evolve; they anchor us, yet allow us freedom for manoeuvre; they underpin our development but do not impede progress.

The values of the National Health Service

The values of general practice cannot be separated from those of the service in which it operates. Since its inception in 1948 the NHS has aspired to provide a comprehensive range of defined high-quality services, free at the point of delivery, funded out of general taxation. There are exceptions, such as prescription and dental charges, but the spirit of this value is still retained. For general practice it means that we provide a service without a consultation or attendance fee: access is not moderated by the ability to pay.

The NHS removed financial barriers to access in order to ensure that it met the health needs of all the people. Some groups have greater needs: the deprived, the elderly, the chronically ill, the mentally ill and children. In more recent times, the desire to address health inequalities has become more important,[10,11] an ideal in which general practice has a key role to play.

Another underlying, but more recently expressed,[2,12] value of the NHS concerns delivering a patient-centred healthcare service. Healthcare must be a partnership with patients and the NHS should be accountable to all citizens, not just a vocal minority. One dimension of this, some might say given over-emphasis of late, is access to the health services. Access must be appropriate, prioritised according to need and equitable – irrespective of geography (especially rural and remote areas), age, sex, ethnicity etc.

Underpinning the NHS and its care should be a bedrock of trust. When patients are ill, or think they are ill, they want to see a doctor who they can trust. Trust is based on the patient's knowledge of their doctor and their clinical and interpersonal skills, and their attitudes. All patients must be cared for by doctors and nurses who are competent and trustworthy, and who are properly accountable for their actions. This trust should also extend to trust between health professionals and the state as their employer, manager and political leader. If trust is diminished – by patients, society, health professionals and managers – then healthcare suffers.

Teamwork is now an essential feature of the British healthcare system, especially in prevention and chronic disease management. Good teams share collective responsibility within a culture of quality improvement and personal development, and teamwork is now a core value of the NHS.

These then are the values of the context in which general practice in Britain exists. They are shared by GPs and are implicit in their working practices.

General practice is not only a main vehicle for expressing and achieving these values, but it has values of its own.

These start with the belief that primary care is an essential feature of an efficient and effective healthcare system. We also believe that general practice and GPs have a unique and important contribution to make to primary care and the NHS. Flexibility in professional boundaries may change some working practices, but the vital central role of a GP cannot be substituted by others. From this we argue that increased investment in primary care, including general practice, will yield better patient outcomes with more efficient use of resources. These assumptions will be tested one by one.

The importance of primary care

From Barbara Starfield's seminal work on international comparisons[13-16] and work by Fry and Horder,[17] it is clear that the more primary care orientation there is in a healthcare system the:

- higher the patient satisfaction with the healthcare system
- lower the overall expenditure on healthcare
- better the population health indicators
- fewer prescribed drugs are taken per head of population.

Why should this be? In British primary care, which is admired throughout the world,[8] we have some valued features that may account for this (*see* Box 5.1). For these reasons we need strong, vibrant primary care in the British NHS.

Box 5.1   The features of British primary care that determine its valuable contribution to the NHS

- The registered list ensures continuity of care, a lifelong record and a family and population approach to healthcare.
- Prevention is intrinsic to the skills and roles of British primary care. Immunisation rates are high, uptake of cervical cytology is a great success story and lifestyle advice is common and opportunistically linked to illness episodes when it is known to be most effective. Screening is now part of everyday general practice in Britain.
- Most patients with a common chronic disease – asthma, hypertension, diabetes, ischaemic heart disease, osteoarthritis – are managed exclusively in primary care.

continued

- The gatekeeper role ensures that those who need access to high technology care or second opinions can receive it. When appropriate, patients are managed in primary care and when referral is indicated the patient sees the appropriate specialist. We protect people from over-medicalisation and exposure to iatrogenic risk.
- Primary care is close to patients, close to the needs of individuals and communities and can ensure the best use of health service resources. The increasing involvement of GPs in public health, commissioning and the response to health inequalities has been positive for the NHS and the health of our nation.

The importance of general practice

There are over 36 000 GP principals in the UK, with an average list size of just over 1800 registered patients. Although the average list size for each principal is falling slightly in historical trends, the number of consultations per unrestricted principal is rising. Since 1984, the number has risen by nearly 800 per year, to 8978 consultations in 1996. This means that principals in general practice perform 324 million consultations a year. When those with non-principals are included, the number rises to about 350 million consultations with GPs per year.

On average, females visit their GP six times a year, and males four times, with an average number of consultations being almost exactly five per year. Both children and the elderly consult more frequently than other age groups. Those under five years old consult on average seven times a year as, also, do those aged over 65, compared to three times for those aged between 16 and 44.

A total of 78% of people in England and Wales consulted their GP at least once during the year 1991/92. The General Household Survey in 1998 found that 14% of people had visited their GP in the previous 14 days. When patients visit the surgery to see a doctor, 87% see their GP or a principal partner, as opposed to a locum, an assistant or a GP registrar. The patient's GP or a partner at the practice carries out 82% of home visits.

Patient satisfaction rates with GP consultations are often very high. The NHS Executive's *National Survey of NHS Patients*[18] reported: 'Most [people who had consulted their GP in the previous 12 months] had favourable views of their GP services. In general, most patients felt that their GPs took their opinions seriously, were easy to understand and kept them well informed about their condition or treatment. 79% considered that their GP knew which treatment was best and 84% that their GP made the right diagnosis most or all of the time.' Despite the complexity, importance and emotional context of GP consultations, they generate less than 5000 formal complaints – one for every 70 000 consultations.

The care of children forms a significant part of the GP's and primary health-care team's workload. Patients aged 15 and under comprise 20% of the average GP's list. Care of the under-fours in particular constitutes a considerable part of the workload of a GP. They consult their GP more often and have more home visits than any other age group except the elderly. The vast majority of children aged 15 and under receive all their medical care from a GP. The rate of referral to hospital (both in- and outpatients) for those aged under 15 is 93 per 1000 consultations, or around 9%.

The 1998 General Household Survey[19] found that in the two weeks before interview, 18% of the under-fives and 9% of 5–15-year-olds had consulted an NHS GP in the 14 days before interview. Figure 5.1 shows where these consultations took place.

Table 5.1 shows that that the vast majority of GPs run effective childhood immunisation programmes. In most cases of failure to immunise more than 70% of children, there are societal explanations.

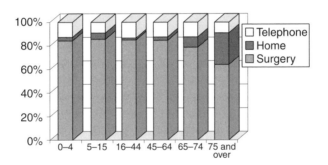

Figure 5.1   Consultations with a GP in the 14 days before interview, by age and site of consultation.[19]

Table 5.1   Target achievements, October 1998, England[20]

	Number	%
Childhood immunisation		
Those achieving 90%	22 991	84
Those achieving 70%	2711	10
Total	25 762	95
Pre-school booster		
Those achieving 90%	22 099	81
Those achieving 70%	3815	14
Total	25 914	95

Figures may not add exactly due to rounding.

Ninety-four per cent of unrestricted principals in England and Wales are on the child health surveillance list. The figures for Scotland and Northern Ireland are 78% and 92% respectively.

The over-65s comprise almost 15% of the average GP's list and the over-75s represent nearly 7%. The 1998 General Household Survey found that 86% of all contacts were managed only in general practice without referral to the wider primary care team, social care or secondary care. In the two weeks before interview, 18% of over-65s had consulted a GP as had 21% of the over-75s. This compares to 13% of those aged between 16 and 44 who had consulted in the two weeks before interview.[19]

From this analysis it can be seen that GPs are undertaking the lion's share of NHS medical work and achieving a high level of patient satisfaction. The GP, as a key part of primary care, is clearly an essential element in the wider health service.

The extent to which a GP's work can be done by others

Primary healthcare is central to the NHS, often determining access to and usage of other services. The integration of all health services – with more communication and less overlap between general practice, out-of-hours arrangements, community nursing, community psychiatric services, hospital outreach, ambulance and acute trusts, especially accident and emergency (A&E) – needs to be improved. The links between social care, including the voluntary provision of health and social care, and the health service are still rudimentary.

Modern general practice is team based and this will increase. The roles of all primary care team members, including GPs, will evolve, for example with enhanced nurse roles such as nurse prescribing. The role of community pharmacists within primary care teams should also be developed.[21]

However, flexibility of roles must take into account core competencies, the most appropriate carer and efficiency. In terms of efficiency, as nurses take on more complex roles such as those undertaken by a nurse practitioner, their consultation duration may extend to over 15 minutes. Extended roles for nurses carry opportunity costs in the erosion of traditional nursing skills that are highly valued by patients and by nurses' professional colleagues.

Flexibility in roles must not just be within individual practices, teams and primary care groups or trusts. It must include a flexibility to provide the correct care for each population's characteristics of geography, demography, ethnicity, culture and socio-economics. The same solutions cannot be applied universally, but variations need to be justified on the basis of the needs of that population, and care must be taken to ensure that every citizen has access to the full range of healthcare professional expertise.

However, these developments must be seen in context. The GP offers the NHS an important range of key attributes and skills. These key attributes include the deployment of complex clinical skills, flexibility, demand management and continuity of care. I will look at each in turn.

Complex clinical skills are the key prerogative of GPs. A GP is presented with the full range of symptoms, signs and histories in the physical, psychological and social domains. Dealing with these needs high-level knowledge, the ability to tolerate uncertainty, the skill to create a safe, effective but not unnecessarily complex management plan and high-level communication skills. While a protocol can offer guidance in the management of uncomplicated cases, most patients are not uncomplicated and many have extensive co-morbidity: angina, hypertension and depression, for example. The capacity to deploy these skills in a short, ten-minute consultation requires a breadth of biomedical and psychosocial knowledge to be matched to the enormous variety of patient presentations. Many come with 'metaphorical' symptoms that need to be unwrapped to reveal the underlying problem. For others, a misinterpretation of the significance of their symptoms can lead to either inappropriate long-term adoption of the sick role or delayed reaction to the early signs of important illness. The complexity of this role, at the interface between perceived illness and disease, must not be underestimated. It is a role for which nurses are not trained. GPs are recruited from the most able school leavers and then intensively trained for nine years. The complexity of the GP's role demands these attributes and is supported by the GP's perceived therapeutic authority.

Flexibility is a hallmark of the personal care delivered by a GP. GPs reformulate their care to meet the needs of individual patients as they evolve, developing roles to suit the needs of patients. This flexibility is the fundamental key to the high quality and high reputation of most general practice. It offers personally tailored care, including the right access to the right parts of the health service when appropriate. Formulaic, protocol-driven care can undermine patient autonomy within the consultation.

Demand management results from GPs empowering patients to take responsibility for their own care when appropriate; from identifying the right routes through the primary and secondary care services and from taking increasing responsibility for complex patient care in general practice.

Continuity of care is highly prized by patients. Seeing a doctor who knows the patient and remembers key events in the life of that patient and the family, who will be there subsequently when required and who takes a longer-term view of care and its outcomes is an important feature of primary care. Continuity has been shown to reduce use of secondary care services and to improve patient satisfaction. Of course, GPs take holidays, retire and move on; not all patients see 'their' GP.

Continuity is supported by four crucial features. Firstly the lifetime clinical record is retained in general practice. The GP is, at present, its guardian, although in time we will see the advent of patient-held and patient-involved records. This record is the key to efficient and safe healthcare delivery. Second, the GP takes a population perspective, with health needs assessment, health inequalities and commissioning being addressed. Next, advocacy on behalf of individual patients, groups of patients and whole communities is a key skill that requires a variety of skills, an overview of the health and social system, the ability to detect and address inequalities and an involvement in commissioning. Good advocacy is based on a shared understanding, which in turn is greatly facilitated by continuity. And lastly, continuity requires taking responsibility. Teamworking is now a key feature of general practice, but the GP continues to take responsibility long after social workers, physiotherapists and practice nurses have finished work.

Conclusion

In this chapter I have looked at those features of general practice that can be described as core values. These have been placed in the wider NHS context, but all healthcare systems need a vibrant primary care system to be cost-effective. The contribution of general practice to the work and working of the NHS is enormous, and without general practice demand, inappropriate care and costs would escalate while many health outcomes would drop.

Within general practice I have identified a range of attributes that distinguish our work. These are highly valued by patients. We are, in essence, the most valued health professional close to the lives of people in this country. We deliver high-quality personal and continuing care, advocating for individuals and groups, and striving, alongside colleagues in primary care, to achieve quality and quantity of life-years.

References

1   Secretary of State for Health and Social Services (1989) *Working for Patients*. Department of Health, London.

2   Secretary of State for Health (2000) *The NHS Plan. A Plan for Investment, A Plan for Reform*. The Stationery Office, London.

3   Secretary of State for Health (2000) *The NHS Plan. A Plan for Pharmacy*. The Stationery Office, London.

4   Speech by Rt Hon Alan Milburn MP, Secretary of State for Health, to the CNO Conference on *Patient Involvement – Public Confidence*, November 2001.

5   British Medical Association (2002) *New GMS Contract*. BMA, London.

6   Department of Health (2002) *Appraisal for General Practitioners Working in the NHS*. DoH, London.

7   Department of Health (2001) *Shifting the Balance of Power: the next steps*. DoH, London.

8   De Maeseneer J, Hjortdahl P and Starfield B (2000) Fix what's wrong, not what's right, with general practice in Britain. *BMJ*. **320**: 1616–17.

9   Royal College of General Practitioners (1972) *The Future General Practitioner: learning and teaching*. BMJ Books, London.

10 Variations Subgroup of the Chief Medical Officer's Health of the Nation Working Group (1995) *Variations in health: what can the Department of Health and the NHS do?* Department of Health, London.

11 Secretary of State for Health (1999) *Saving Lives: our healthier nation*. Department of Health, London.

12 Department of Health (2001) *The National Service Framework for Diabetes: standards*. DoH, London.

13 Starfield B (1994) Is primary care essential? *Lancet*. **344**: 1129–33.

14 Starfield B and Oliver T (1999) Primary care in the United States and its precarious future. *Health and Social Care in the Community*. **7** (5): 315–23.

15 Starfield B (1998) *Primary Care: balancing health needs, services and technology*. Oxford University Press, New York.

16 Starfield B (1997) The future of primary care in a managed care era. *International Journal of Health Services*. **27**: 687–96.

17 Fry J and Horder J (1995) *Primary Health Care in an International Context*. Nuffield Provincial Hospitals Trust, London.

18 NHS Executive (1999) *National Survey of NHS Patients*. NHSE, Leeds.

19 Office for National Statistics (Social Survey Division) (2000) *Living in Britain: Results from the 1998 General Household Survey*. The Stationery Office, London.

20 Department of Health Statistical Bulletin 1999/13 (2000) *Statistics for General Medical Practitioners in England: 1988–1998*. DoH, London.

21 Royal College of General Practitioners (2000) *The RCGP's View on the Future Role of the Pharmacist in Primary Care*. RCGP, London.

CHAPTER 6

The value of general practice to the public

Patricia Wilkie

Introduction

My first memory of general practice was attending, as a young teenager, a three-doctor practice in a central Scottish town with a population of less than 2000. At that time there was both an appointment system and an open surgery. I do not remember any difficulty in seeing the doctor of choice. I do remember the doctor's cheery face appearing in the waiting room to call in the next patient, and I remember the consideration given to me and my problem, however trivial it may have seemed to the doctor. Consultations always included questions such as 'And how are things at home? And at school?' and were asked with a smile and a raised eyebrow! Some 20 years later, and in my capacity as chair of a voluntary organisation, I accompanied a lady, whose husband and both adult children had Huntington's disease, to discuss with her general practitioner, at his request, problems relating to that illness. This was my former GP now working in a socially deprived area of a large city. He said that he did not have other patients on his list with the same illness and that he wanted both to find out from the family what were the problems facing the patients and their family and to work with them to provide the appropriate care and support. It was wonderful to find the same doctor working in a very different environment but still offering what is now described as patient-centred care, and with great compassion. [Dr Walter Galloway, 1923–2001.]

Background

The society in which patients and doctors live affects the relationship between them. Fifty years ago when the RCGP was founded, the Conservatives had won the election of 1951 and Churchill was again prime minister, Queen Elizabeth II had recently come to the throne, rationing of some commodities was still in existence and the NHS was already being used by 95% of the population.[1] The war in Korea from 1951–53 had diverted resources from much needed social investment and national service was still compulsory. Contemporary reports suggested that the 'gravest weaknesses in the NHS were due to the low level of capital expenditure'. In January 1952, Harry Crookshank, the new Minister of Health, proposed certain charges in the NHS, thus breaking with the underlying philosophy of the NHS that healthcare should be free at the point of delivery. These charges included one shilling (5p) on each prescription dispensed and £1 for dental treatment. However, what the patients in the study by Brotherston and Chave,[2] who found that on one housing estate 99 prescriptions were issued for every 100 consultations, thought of the new charges is unknown.

In 1952 patients consulted 'their doctor' in premises located in streets near where they lived. The doctors worked in small practices and often, by 2003 standards, from modest consulting rooms. The waiting room was often the 'front room' of the doctor's house. Many practices worked with an open system for consultations. Appointment systems were less common. Few practices had nurses working with them. And there was still a popularly held belief that GPs and their patients knew one another, immortalised by Will Fyffe's song of Dr MacGregor:

> Dr MacGregor and his wee black bag
> Known at every cottage door throughout the countryside
> There is not a bed he has not sat beside ...

By contrast, in 2003 most GPs work from health centres alongside other health professionals. Health centres may not be so conveniently situated for everyone and may require patients to use a car or public transport to visit. However, with the new working environment many patients now have a choice not only of which doctor to consult, but whether to consult a doctor, a nurse or another health professional. In addition, patients can receive advice and information by phone from NHS Direct and visit a walk-in clinic for help and treatment previously often given by a GP.

Over the last 50 years the treatments available to patients have changed. From the perspective of the patient some of these changes are important. For example, more and better drug therapies for people with such illnesses as diabetes, certain cancers and cystic fibrosis have resulted in improvement in clinical outcomes as well as in the quality of life. There are also other changes in that patients may not need to remain in hospital as more procedures can now be carried out in day surgery. Furthermore, patients with problems previously only looked after in hospital may now be discharged from hospital to be cared for in the community. Such changes create challenges for GPs and patients alike, and for many patients make the role of, and the relationship with, the GP even more important.

Sources of information about patients' views

What do patients think of general practice and their GP? Fifty years ago academic medicine was already well established but clinical studies rarely considered the views of the patient. It was not until the 1960s that there were increasing numbers of scholarly articles highlighting different aspects of medical inter-actions from the perspective of the patient, mainly from the relatively new discipline of medical sociology. For example, the work of Anne Cartwright[3] highlighted the importance of information for patients. Other studies opened the debate about power in the doctor–patient relationship, the nature of the consultation, the use of language in the consultation, the influence of social class on health and illness, and definitions of illness.[4] Jefferys[5] found that patients in the 1970s seldom criticised the clinical judgement or technical competence of their doctor, but they were concerned that their GP was 'not so warm or friendly as they would like' and that 'they had difficulty in telling their GP all that he or she should know about them and their condition'.

It was not until 1967 that the General Medical Council (GMC), and in 1968 the Royal Commission on Medical Education, recommended that all medical students should pursue some study of sociology. However, it was with the rise of the consumer movement and self-help groups in the 1960s that the public, the profession and the governments of the day began to hear about what changes patients and users of services would like to see.[6] In the 1960s there was a new generation that questioned established traditions. This generation had both the ability and the confidence to set up organisations and press for change. Few of these organisations were solely concerned with general practice but the principles they eschewed applied to most medical specialities, including general practice.

In 1961, the National Association for the Welfare of Children in Hospital (NAWCH) was founded as a result of the concern of the founders that the mes-sage of the Platt report of 1959 that children needed regular and continuing contact with their parents was being ignored. NAWCH campaigned for the uni-versal adoption of unrestricted visiting in children's wards and for the provision of accommodation to enable mothers to stay in hospital with their child. In the same year, the National Childbirth Trust (NCT) and the Association for the Improvement of Maternity Services were founded by women who wanted to be involved as partners in their antenatal care and in the planning of the birth. What seemed logical to women was often ridiculed by professionals. In 1963, the Patients' Association was founded as a result of a letter to the *Observer* newspaper from a lady who alleged that she had been the subject of medical experimen-tation during her pregnancy. The early work of the Patients' Association focused on patients' rights to refuse to be used in the teaching of medical students and the part that patients played in medical research. The Patients' Association has since expanded to lobby for patients' interests in healthcare.

More recently a collaborative study by the NHS Confederation and the Long-term Medical Condition Alliance[7] found that in general patients were very supportive of GPs, but that there was a feeling that health services had become more impersonal and the suggestion that the development of new, larger surgeries involving many GPs may make the opportunity for patients to build a quality relationship with a GP unrealistic.

For the future, individual practices are now encouraged to survey the views of patients. Indeed it will be a requirement in the new GP contract and perhaps for revalidation for GPs to have carried out a patient survey. However, the challenge for the future is for more practices to involve patients in the design of studies, thus ensuring that questions meaningful to patients will be asked. The emergence of the critical consumer, by no means peculiar to healthcare, has changed the relationship between some doctors and their patients.

Aspects of general practice valued by patients

The job description for a GP, and defined by the RCGP in 1969, states 'the general practitioner is a doctor who provides personal, primary and continuing medical care to individuals and families'. It is these attributes of continuing and personal care that have continued to be appreciated by patients. For example, Smith and Armstrong[8] showed that patients' preferences for criteria of good healthcare (and these were criteria originated by patients) were:

- doctors who listen
- usually being able to see the same doctor
- doctors who sort out problems.

However, it is interesting to note that 35 years earlier, Richard Titmuss,[9] in a paper presented to the annual meeting of the BMA, suggested that patients would increasingly be looking for:

- scientific expertise
- personal interest and psychological understanding
- continuity of care
- right to choose whether to be treated at home or in hospital.

Titmuss includes two elements – scientific expertise and choice – that are not mentioned in the later Smith and Armstrong work,[8] but are features that are now most highly regarded by patients.

Martin Roland, in his 1998 Mackenzie lecture,[10] identified the following as aspects of general practice that patients now hope to find:

- availability and accessibility

- technical competence
- continuity of care
- communication skills, including providing time to explore patients' needs, listening, explaining, giving information and sharing decisions
- humaneness, caring, supportiveness and trust.

These attributes will now be discussed in more detail.

Availability and time

At the beginning of the twenty-first century, time for doctors and patients alike has become a most precious commodity. The pressures on us all are such that we want instant solutions to our problems whether as a patient or as a carer, and in many circumstances we need the help of our GP to diagnose, treat or refer appropriately. Consultation rates with GPs are rising. It is therefore understand-able that because of the increase in patient, professional and administrative demands on general practice over the last 50 years, different systems have been introduced to manage availability. These have included fewer home visits, the development of nurse-led specialist clinics, telephone access to either a GP or other health professional, the widespread use of deputising services and systems where no appointments can be made more than 48 hours in advance. In addition, the Department of Health from time to time (and usually before major public holidays) issues information about when to consult a doctor and how to treat self-limiting viral infections.

The consultation time is also an important factor and the profession is aware of the advantages of a longer consultation for both doctor and patient. There is evidence[11,12] that the quality of the interaction between doctor and patient can have a major influence on health outcomes. However, as Marinker has pointed out,[13] considerable skill is required by both doctor and patient to have quality of interaction in a consultation of around seven minutes.

One of the aims of the RCGP initiative *How to Work with your Doctor*,[14] which itself was a partnership between doctors and lay people, was to give information to patients about the sort of questions they may need to consider before the consultation, including:

- when the person first noticed the symptoms or started feeling ill
- what makes the condition better or worse
- what the pain or problem actually feels like.

Patients can also be encouraged to ask the following questions during the con-sultation:

- What is the cause of the problem?

- How is the problem normally treated?
- What can the patient do about the problem?
- Are there any long-term effects?
- Is there anything that the patient can do to prevent the problem happening again?

The challenge for patients today is to learn how to make the best use of consultation time. Many will need the help of their practitioner to do so.

Technical competence

It is now expected of all professionals that they are competent to do their work and that they keep up to date – and most GPs do so. The RCGP should be proud of the leading role it has taken over the last 50 years in promoting vocational training. However, 50 years ago most patients would have assumed that the doctor would know what the problem was and how best to treat it.[15] It has now become so important that GPs are technically and scientifically competent. Patients discharged from secondary and tertiary sectors on complicated treatment regimens are dependent on the skill of their GP to maintain therapy and to detect when there may be problems. In these circumstances patients have to trust their GP.

However, technical competence does not mean that the GP knows all the answers. At the present time the public have become increasingly aware that doctors do not know everything and some may not have kept up to date. The public are also beginning to realise what many individual patients have already come to understand – that medicine is not an exact science. In contrast with 50 years ago, patients do not expect their GP to know about all illnesses and respect doctors who know the limits of their own knowledge and when and from where to seek advice. Patients need their GP to make an appropriate and timely referral, and trust and rely on them to do so.

I became very aware of this aspect of general practice when, as an undergraduate student in 1969, I spent one day per week for a term with the Lipetz practice (Drs Sam and Julius Lipetz) in inner-city Edinburgh. Patients came from either the socially deprived east end or from amongst staff and students of Edinburgh University. Referral letters were frequently written in the presence of the patient. They were succinct yet appropriately detailed and were very highly regarded by consultants. A consequence of this was that the initial visit to hospital was easier for the patient. It was not unusual for Dr Sam Lipetz, who long outlived the premature death of his younger brother, to inform the patient that he would like to consult a reference or a colleague before making a decision. These GPs were much respected by patients and colleagues alike. I was privileged to have worked with them and to have subsequently been their patient.

Continuity of care

Earlier and contemporary studies have all shown that patients value continuity of care, a doctor who knows them and a doctor who listens. At the beginning of our period individual GPs did offer continuity of care. That rare breed of single-handed doctors, those in small practices and those with personal lists can perhaps more easily provide continuity of care. However, patients now have a choice of which doctor to consult. Younger patients, those with a self-limiting condition or those in a hurry may not mind which doctor they see, making continuity of care from the perspective of patients much more difficult. But when patients have a chronic illness or perhaps as patients get older, continuity of care and a personal interest become even more valued.

In larger practices it is arguable that it is not the individual doctor who offers continuity of care, but the practice. Members of the practice may be satisfied that there are good methods of communication between staff, and within the practice good systems for receiving messages and recording reports and letters, all of which are necessary to provide continuity of care. Many patients will be unaware of the relevance of continuity of care. These patients see different doctors, different receptionists on different occasions and come with different problems. In these circumstances patients can feel isolated. The challenge for the profession is how to maintain quality and in particular how to maintain continuity of care. The challenge for patients is to learn how to work with the system and to make appropriate decisions about with whom and when to consult.

Sharing decisions and communication

In this chapter many differences for both doctors and patients over the last 50 years of general practice have been described. But it is also clear that over this period patients have continued to lay great importance on personal care, technical competence and having a doctor who listens. Fifty years ago the great majority of patients accepted without question the advice of, and treatment recommended by, their doctor: 'Doctor knew best.' Today patient involvement is being encouraged by the government as a way of improving the quality of service in healthcare and in general practice. Patients now expect to be given information about their condition, about the options for treatment and about how their illness can be managed. Some have argued that this desire to be involved in the decisions about our healthcare is peculiar to articulate, middle-class patients. However, according to Coulter and Elwyn,[16] the evidence does not support this, and trials of decision aids to inform patients and to enable them to play a more active role in their care have revealed strong support amongst patients from all social groups.

The success of active involvement of patients in their own care will depend to a great extent on good relationships, good communication and trust between patients and their doctor. This is particularly important when decisions involve uncertainty and/or discussions about risk. Many individual patients have already come to understand that medicine is not an exact science. These are not easy concepts for doctors and patients to talk about.

The challenge for GPs is to accept that most patients can and do want to be involved in their own care. The challenge for patients is to learn to work with their GP in shared decision making.

The above discussion concerns patients' involvement in their own care. The government also encourages public involvement in health policy. Twenty years ago the RCGP established a Patient Liaison Group (PLG) to assist the College by bringing to its attention concerns of patients and the wider public about general practice. At that time the College was unique amongst the medical Royal Colleges in establishing a PLG. It has taken several years for the majority of the other Royal Colleges to begin to follow the example of the RCGP. In the last few years the majority of the medical Royal Colleges have established PLGs based on the RCGP model. The group is composed of almost equal numbers of lay and medical members. The opportunity for debate between medical and lay colleagues in an atmosphere of trust and respect is unusual. Topics of concern raised by the PLG have often become topics of major debate in the College. The advantage of the PLG discussing a particular topic is that the deliberation may be broader than if doctors on their own discussed the subject. The presence of lay members can provide credibility at a time when partnership between doctors and lay people is being encouraged. There is now a lay member from the PLG on most of the main committees of the Council of the RCGP and the lay chairperson of the PLG attends the Council Executive Committee (CEC) in addition to Council. The College was inspired in establishing the PLG so early and in encouraging and allowing lay people to be involved in policy decisions.

Humaneness

In this chapter, I think that it is appropriate to include personal views. Reference has already been made to the suggestion that in the 1950s most patients knew their GP and vice versa. Dr John and Dr Vina Wilkie, my parents-in-law, were in partnership in general practice in Lancaster for over 30 years. I often observed the little smile, or the inclination of the head, or sometimes even a wave as patients from the practice were recognised. There were also little kindnesses when they learned of the death of a patient or troubles in a family. There was humanity in their actions. A very different personality was my uncle, Dr Robbie McGregor. Shortly before he retired I walked with him along the main street of Hawick, in the Scottish borders, where Robbie had been a GP for many years. He seemed to know everyone by name and the members of the family. Underneath the rather blustery exterior there was kindliness and a real interest in his fellow human beings.

Conclusion

In this chapter many of the challenges facing contemporary general practice have been explored. The changing relationships between patients and their GP are indeed a challenge for both patients and doctors. The values that patients see as important in their GP are also the values that are shared with the profession. With the object of the RCGP 'to encourage, foster and maintain the highest possible standards in general medical practice' patients and their GPs can surely look forward with optimism.

References

1   Marwick A (1970) *Britain in the Century of Total War*. Penguin, Harmondsworth.

2   Brotherston J and Chave S (1956) General practice on a new housing estate. *British Journal of Preventive and Social Medicine*. **10**: 200.

3   Cartwright A (1967) *Patients and their Doctors*. Routledge–Kegan Paul, London.

4   Tuckett D (1976) *An Introduction to Medical Sociology*. Tavistock Publications, London.

5   Jefferys M (1977) What are health services for: whom do they serve? *New Universities Quarterly*. **30** (2): 181–92.

6   Wilkie P (1999) The patient perspective. In: Sims J (ed.) *Primary Health Care Sciences*. Whurr Publishers, London.

7   Lewthwaite R and Joule N (1997) Patients Influencing Purchasers. Report of a project sponsored by the Long-Term Medical Condition Alliance. NHS Confederation, Birmingham.

8   Smith CH and Armstrong D (1989) Comparison of criteria derived by government and patients for evaluating general practitioner services. *BMJ*. **299** (6697): 494–6.

9   Titmuss RM (1968) *Commitment to Welfare*. Allen & Unwin, London.

10 Roland M (1999) James Mackenzie lecture 1998: Quality and efficiency: enemies or partners? *British Journal of General Practice*. **49** (439): 140–3.

11 Kaplan SH, Greenfield S and Ware JE (1989) Assessing the effects of physician–patient interactions on the outcomes of chronic disease. *Medical Care*. **27** (3): 110–27.

12 Horder J and Moore JT (1990) The consultation and health outcomes. *British Journal of General Practice*. **40**: 442–3.

13 Marinker M (1997) *From Compliance to Concordance: achieving shared goals in medicine taking*. Royal Pharmaceutical Society/Merck, Sharpe & Dohme, London.

14 Royal College of General Practitioners (1997) *How to Work with your Doctor*. Report of a project of the RCGP's Patients' Liaison Group. RCGP, London.

15 McGregor RM (1969) *The Work of the Family Doctor*. Livingstone, Edinburgh.

16 Coulter A and Elwyn G (2002) What do patients want from high-quality general practice and how do we involve them in improvement? *British Journal of General Practice*. **52** (Suppl.): S22–S25.

CHAPTER 7

Celebrating the study of the doctor–patient relationship

Sally Hull

To write prescriptions is easy, but to come to an understanding with people is hard.

Franz Kafka, a country doctor

Morning surgery has started at my practice in east London. Six doctors have full lists with patients booked at ten-minute intervals, two nurses are running clinics. Telephones are busy and the triage nurse, who assesses everyone asking for a same-day appointment, has ten to call back so far. Halfway through the morning Mohammed Aziz comes in:

> He is a 44-year-old man from Pakistan, grey-haired and dapper, who has chosen to see me although registered with my partner. An infrequent attender, I have seen him twice, both times for a painful right elbow which prevents him working as a waiter. On the second occasion I injected this as a tennis elbow, but remember predicting to myself that this would not help his symptoms.
>
> As he came in today he said he was no better and fell silent. In the reflective space between us I noticed his stillness, and also that he was wearing a smart white shirt and tie. Something tragic could be felt in the dissonance between his behaviour and the complaint. I asked him about his work before he left Bangladesh. Over the next few minutes he told me how, fearing persecution, he had to leave a flourishing business, and his family, and come to London where he works as a waiter. The depth of his lonely separation from his wife and children, and the disappointing course his recent life has taken, was easily conveyed. As he opened the door to leave he asked for my support for their entry application.

The doctor–patient relationship is largely enacted through face-to-face consultations, and encounters such as this form the core work of general practice.

British general practice has provided a major contribution to the study of the encounter between doctors and patients. Historically this has developed from the core attributes of general practice: the registered patient list, personal continuity of care and open access to the doctor regardless of the nature of the problem. The contract in general practice is to a person, not to a particular age group or to a specific therapeutic technique. This study of the encounter between people in medical settings has had important effects on the identity of the discipline, on the nature of training and research for practice, and has also had widespread effects on teaching in hospital medicine. As we think about the significance of general practice-based primary care in this country over the last 50 years, I have chosen three approaches to the study of the doctor–patient encounter, which are illustrated in the account of the man with a painful elbow.

Those of us who have had the privilege of vocational training, and have been encouraged to formulate our diagnoses in physical, psychological and social dimensions, will have difficulty looking back from our perspective to recall the importance of the shift in focus of the 'clinical gaze'[1] which occurred in general practice in the 1950s to 1960s. This shift in the nature of what constituted the material for study was articulated most prominently by Michael Balint in his case discussion work with groups of general practitioners.[2] The doctor has come into view within the clinical encounter. What the doctor observes and feels about the patient has become part of the clinical case material. In the case illustration the doctor uses an empathic identification with the patient, and then is able to reflect on that brief 'flash' of feeling and use it as a cue to change the nature of the discussion. This approach can be seen as a reversal of the direction, prominent in hospital medicine, which had progressively objectified the patient and presented the clinical case as a technical pathological puzzle.

The second theme is based on work stimulated by social scientists which has looked critically at social roles within the encounter, and also at the behavioural building blocks of the consultation. This has fostered a dynamic development of skills-based consultation teaching, consultation theory, and has stimulated empirical work which has begun to identify elements of the doctor–patient relationship which affect clinical outcomes.

The third theme is the question of the story, and how GPs stand at the intersection of illness expressed in physical symptoms and life story. How does our response to this position at the crossroads affect the development of the illness? The exploration of the consultation as story and the different roles that the study of narrative can have in enlightening the clinical encounter developed momentum in the 1980s as narrative-based medicine.

Exploration of the doctor–patient relationship

At the time that Michael Balint[2] started his exploratory groups in the 1950s, much of general practice was in a depressed state. Many GPs had little in the way of facilities or training to do a job which was perplexing, with much of the content of clinical encounters falling outside the categories of technical medicine which were in ascendancy in the training hospitals. This is acutely captured by David Morrell, who entered general practice in 1957:[3]

> The early weeks and months in the consulting room were confusing, and I was filled with feelings of guilt. The knowledge and skills acquired in hospital just did not seem relevant to the many problems I encountered.... I was not aware of the political battles over general practice at the time, but was simply conscious of my own inadequacies and people's constant demand for care.

The work that was done by Michael and Enid Balint provided a meeting place for the ideas of psychoanalysis and the material of general practice, with the aim of studying the everyday work of general practice and exploring some of the psychological aspects of what GPs actually did. The groups had both a training and a research agenda and required a prolonged commitment of weekly meetings, usually for about three years. Initially the agenda was set by Michael Balint, the data to be examined being the nature of the interaction as seen by the doctor. This quote illustrates how the doctor was to be brought into the field of vision:[2]

> The events that I wanted to get hold of could be observed only by the doctor himself; the presence of a third person, however tactful and objective, would inevitably destroy the ease and intimacy of the atmosphere. Such a third person would see only an imitation, perhaps a very good imitation, but never the real thing.

The group was used as a way of capturing, describing and amplifying the details of the doctor–patient relationship revealed to the group.[4] Much of the case material came from troubled or stuck relationships developed over years of contact.

One of the ideas brought from dynamic psychotherapy, which informed the group method, was that some aspects of relationships which may be problematic for the patient could be reflected within the relationship with their doctor.

The leader in the group, initially an analyst but latterly GPs with training in group leadership, helps the group to stay focused on the relationship, the contract being that the material discussed will not stray too far into the world of the patient or too far into the personal or intra-psychic world of the doctor.

With the shift in paradigm started by this controversial change in the direction of the clinical gaze, many aspects of the work of general practice were brought into view which previously had been unobserved, part of the tacit clinical behaviour of doctors, or perhaps thought not to be worth serious study. The work done within Balint groups is an example of case-based qualitative research which began to identify and describe some of the clinical uses of the doctor–patient relationship.[5–7] This method has been described as the only true ethnographic research method that general practice has evolved.[8]

Many of the findings and pithy descriptions which were the output of the research groups have become embedded in the everyday language of general practice. The idea of the doctor–patient relationship itself, along with the proposition that it may at times be a mirror of other relationships that are of importance in the patient's life. The value of a continuing relationship between the doctor and patient, rich with shared information and intimacy leading to trust, was described as a 'mutual investment company' in which both parties have invested and both can draw interest. The idea of the doctor's 'apostolic function' which described how doctors more or less consciously tend to impose their views and expectations on the patient on how to behave when ill. The idea of the 'doctor as drug', which had of course long been around in other guises, but the contribution of the Balint method was to see the need for this to be opened up to understand the variety of ways in which this drug can be used both in diagnostic and therapeutic ways.[5,9,10]

These ideas have had an influence which spread far beyond the small circle of doctors who worked in training or research groups. Tudor Hart[11] identified three aspects of the work that Balint did with GPs which had an important effect on the development of general practice as an independent discipline.

First, GPs gained the confidence to examine both the clinical and the organisational content of their work. Second, they began to see that it was the training that was wrong rather than what was presented to them in clinical encounters, and that they would have to take control themselves to develop the theories and tools which were necessary to provide effective practice. Third, he demonstrated that to provide effective care it is necessary to look beyond the immediate demands of the encounter. This influence can be traced from the original formulation of the training required for effective practice in *The Future General Practitioner: learning and teaching*[12] to the continued inclusion of case discussion groups based on Balint group ideas in most vocational training schemes today.

There continues to be international interest in case-based discussion groups both for training and for research, although currently there is far more activity in European countries and the USA than in the UK.[13] Recent research monographs have looked at how doctors can remain sensitive to the surprises which develop in their relationships with patients, and have studied the defences that doctors practise in their encounters.[7,14] There are also some examples of how GPs have led the way in using their observations of the doctor–patient relationship to illuminate aspects of their work with patients.

An example is a case series on intimacy and terminal care by Gilley.[15] This is a personal reflection on four cases of people with terminal illness requesting visits. It illustrates the link between the expression of physical intimacy and the place of death. Through the cases she illustrates how both overt and covert communication about the past and present experience of intimacy and contact can translate into the most appropriate arrangement for terminal care when they are sensitively observed within the doctor–patient relationship and used for the patient's benefit. Other examples include studies which have attempted to examine the effect of the doctor changing how they behave in the consultation from a sharing to a directive style of consultation.[16,17] The results of these studies suggest that where doctors provide a positive, patient-centred approach, patients will be both more satisfied and enabled to gain control over their symptoms. They may also be less burdened by their symptoms and may use less health service resources.[18]

Do these ideas retain a currency today? A prevailing view among many GPs is that Balint is history, that the work done by the Balints has been superseded by other approaches to the consultation, and that much of the language associated with Balint has become a cliché to be discarded as the terrain is explored anew with the different focus of a new generation. Clearly, much of the influence that Michael Balint had on the context of the discipline of general practice in the 1950s is of historical interest. However, this is quite different from suggesting that the work itself, this particular ethnographic method which the Balints developed of looking at the core work of general practice, is no longer relevant to doctors working today. Closely allied to the view of 'Balint as history' is the view that knowledge proceeds progressively, that one development is eclipsed by another, that an orderly advance through the forests of unknowing can be made. This is rarely true even in the basic sciences, but even less true of knowledge about us which has a tendency to become corrupted or lost and requires an iterative, reflective cycle of exploration. Each new generation has to find afresh what they need to learn through the Balint method. It is a different style of learning to the acquisition of intellectual knowledge, and the need for this can never become outdated.[7]

Tasks and skills: the process of the consultation

The second type of enquiry into the doctor–patient relationship as it is enacted in the consultation is a more reductionist set of questions. These seek to find out about the process of the consultation, about the detailed behaviour of the doctor and what effect this might have upon outcomes such as satisfaction, understanding or concordance with treatment aims.

The growth in studies of the interaction between doctors and patients was greatest in the 1970s and 1980s, when all the social science disciplines participated in a vigorous exploration and challenge to the established notions of the traditional forms of consultation. Other authors have reviewed the literature.[19] I can only identify some of the landmark publications which chart the way that general practice has collaborated, and used the material to develop its own body of consultation theory for reflective practice, training and research.

At the beginning of this period the traditional medical model seemed self-explanatory. History was followed by examination, diagnosis led to treatment. How this was done, the antecedents to the consultation, the language used, the social roles, indeed the entire nature of the interaction with the patient were seen as secondary, part of the bedside manner of the doctor.

As general practice, largely through the activity and development of the RCGP, became a discipline with a specific body of expertise which was to be explored and transmitted during a training period, the consultation itself came under increasing scrutiny.

The verbal behaviour of doctors in consultation was extensively studied by Byrne and Long using audiotapes. They generated the idea of the doctor-centred (based on doctors' knowledge) and patient-centred (including patients' experience) styles of consultation. But perhaps of more importance were their observations on the relative inflexibility of a doctor's preferred style, the tendency to interrupt early, and their observations on dysfunctional consultations where often the doctor had not spent time on clearly identifying the reason for why the patient was there. As the authors stress:[20]

> The doctor is, we say, 'both a product and a prisoner of his medical education' which has made no attempt to provide him with behaviours suited to enable him to cope with psychosocial problems.

This work, in combination with the broad training agenda developed by the RCGP, led to a changed view of what the consultation was for. The traditional brief encounter in which the patient presented symptoms and the doctor gave a treatment was no longer adequate. The restatement of the purpose of the consultation was expressed in the elegant formulation of Stott and Davis (*see* Box 7.1). This uses a four-part framework to describe the potential of each primary care consultation, and expands the professional agenda of general practice by pulling into view aspects of anticipatory care and the management of chronic disease which have since then become essential components of every doctor's work.[21]

The contribution of social sciences has been essential to the development of consultation theory within general practice. Anthropologists have illuminated the nature of therapeutic ritual and medical authority, the difficulties of

---

Box 7.1   The potential of each primary care consultation[21]

A Management of presenting problems	**B** Modification of help-seeking behaviours
C Management of continuing problems	**D** Opportunistic health promotion

communicating across a cultural divide, and have pointed to the cultural gap that may exist between doctors and patients within an ostensibly similar culture, and how this may impede communication.[19,22]

There are two themes from this long and fruitful alliance between sociologists and social psychologists working with general practice which have had a particular impact on understanding the consultation and using it effectively for the benefit of patients. The first is the concept brought from social psychology of health belief models, developed in the context of studies on compliance with medication or advice. This model stresses that the context in which advice is given is important. It encourages the identification of three elements of patients' beliefs and understandings about health and illness, including perceived vulnerability to a condition, the perception of seriousness and a personal weighting of the costs and benefits of action or inaction. The importance of these models is their plasticity, their mutability particularly under the conditions when patients engage in a struggle to understand what is happening to them during the course of illness. Doctors who remain ignorant of their patients' health beliefs will fail to make use of an important arena of dialogue where changes can be negotiated.[23]

The second theme comes from the work of Tuckett, elaborated in his description of the consultation as a meeting between experts: the doctor by his training and experience comes with access to specialist knowledge; the patient on the other hand comes with his past experience and set of ideas about what is happening to him. Both parties form models of what is wrong and what is to be done. These models may be uncertain, and there may be considerable inconsistency between them. A major aim of the consultation must be to have an explicit sharing of these models.[24]

One of the major achievements of work on the consultation in British general practice has been to work with the theory and empirical findings from different disciplines and to integrate them into a pragmatic model of the components of a consultation which can be used for teaching and training. The views of patients are firmly in evidence here as well. What we know from patients is that they want to have more time with their doctors, and that the elements of a good consultation include attention both to effective clinical skills and to communication. A good consultation for the patient is one in which the doctor exhibits a participatory style, that is: listens, appears interested, volunteers explanations and negotiates treatments.[19]

The tasks and skills model of the consultation is built upon a clear view of what the purpose of the consultation is, alongside an exposition of the range of skills and strategies which can be used to achieve each component of the consultation.[25] This model is now a core feature in every vocational training scheme and is embedded in the consultation module for summative assessment as well as the RCGP membership examination. This model and its derivatives have spread widely throughout medicine through their influence on the teaching of communication skills to undergraduates, initially in general practice modules, using role play, video and actors (*see* Box 7.2).

This outlines how general practice, along with other disciplines, has pioneered the exploration of doctor–patient communication. The foundations and tools of the relationship have been identified. But what of the evidence that these attributes have an effect on health outcomes?

Personal doctoring has often rather loosely been subsumed within the phrase 'continuity of care'. But it can be seen to have two elements: the development of a relationship in which the patient feels they know their doctor well, and care given continuously by the same doctor over a long period of time. Longitudinal continuity may imply a personal relationship, but as Freeman has pointed out, seeing the same doctor does not guarantee either a satisfactory or an effective doctor–patient relationship.[26] What matters more is personal continuity, which contains the elements of empathy and personal responsibility and is summed up by the feeling that the patient knows the doctor well. Personal continuity, which is dependent on the effectiveness of communication, can develop over a short – and interrupted – series of consultations. What patients want is a doctor who listens and who sorts out problems. The key factors associated with patient satisfaction are the provision of information, medical skills and interpersonal skills.[27]

These factors have been shown to have benefits for both patients and doctors. Patient enablement – gaining a sense of mastery over their condition – and

---

Box 7.2   The tasks of the consultation[25]

- To find out why the patient has come, including:
  - the nature and history of the problems
  - their aetiology
  - the patient's ideas, concerns and expectations
  - the effects of the problems.
- To consider other problems, including:
  - continuing problems
  - risk factors.
- To choose an appropriate action for each problem with the patient.
- To achieve a shared understanding of the problems with the patient.
- To involve the patient in management, and to encourage appropriate responsibility.
- To use time and resources appropriately
  - in the consultation
  - in the long term.
- To establish or maintain a relationship with the patient which helps to achieve the other tasks.

compliance with medication are improved when the patient feels they know the doctor well.[29,30] Some 75% of patients report having at least one personal GP in a recent Oxfordshire survey, and interestingly 18% report having two. Having a personal doctor–patient relationship was not seen as important for minor illness, but was highly valued by both patients and GPs for more serious conditions and for psychological issues. For these conditions it was valued more than a convenient appointment.[31]

The story and how to understand it

> I would like to advance the argument that a medicine which regards the patient not only as an object but also as a subject continues to exist in general practice.... It persists precisely because the patient refuses to be ill according to the best precepts of modern medical education.[32]

The third way in which general practice has contributed to understanding the doctor–patient relationship is through the study of narrative-based medicine: identifying the story the patient is telling us, and exploring the different levels at which we can understand and respond to this. This attention to the form and function of narrative within medical encounters has grown in significance since the 1980s and is of increasing importance as we grapple with integrating the abstracted information from evidence-based medicine alongside the unique experiences of the individual with us in the consulting room.[28]

Understanding the value of narrative starts with considering it within the diagnostic encounter.[33] A story is the form in which patients express their experience of illness. If the doctor listens for long enough without interruption (on average the doctor interrupts after only 18 seconds, yet if the patient is allowed to proceed the story usually lasts only half a minute) there will also be clues as to some of the ways the patients understand their illness, and how they are incorporating it into their own life narrative. The well-told illness story is also a tool for promoting understanding between doctor and patient, a means of encouraging empathic understanding.

One of the complex tasks for the doctor in the consulting room is to take into account at least two forms of the narrative that are presented to them by the patient. At one level the doctor needs to abstract from the language of the story the parts of the encounter that form a common theme which is peculiar to medicine, the abstracted case history. In the example of the case given at the beginning the case history might be summarised as: 'Pakistani man, aged 44, with pain in the lateral aspect of the right elbow brought on by the repetitive movements of his work as a waiter. Examination shows epicondylitis. Treat with a local steroid injection and refrain from work.'

At the same time the doctor has to hold in mind the individual context surrounding the abstracted story for that patient, which may help to define in what particular way the patient is becoming ill. For the man with the painful arm the contextual narrative is beginning to emerge: we can hear a lonely and disappointed man who feels condemned to work his passage into a new country in a repetitive, meaningless job without even having the support and love of his close family about him.

For much of the time the doctor–patient relationship itself will form a small subplot in a minor episode of the patient's life narrative. But for some individuals the relationship may loom large, and there are a number of occasions when the possibility of understanding comes at a crucial time. General practitioners have been described as the guardians of the interface between illness and disease.[34] The role of the doctor at this particular boundary helps in the process of engaging in a dialogue which may safeguard the patient from the too ready interpretation of illness as disease rather than distress. Or indeed the opposite, to protect patients against their own willingness to accept as a condition of life bodily experiences which require a biomedical solution. The image of the doctor at the boundary is an important one for other aspects of the fulfilment of personal narrative. In the therapeutic process, active listening to the narrative can be potentially therapeutic or palliative and is an example of the doctor's role as a needed witness to the personal story of the patient.[33,35] The biographic role of the doctor has also been described as the hermeneutic function.[34] At times interpretation and assistance in organising the illness story into a coherent whole with the patient is important. Indeed this may be why both doctors and therapists seek in their work with the patient to facilitate an alternative viewpoint, to develop with the patient a more constructive life narrative which makes sense from the patient's point of view.[36]

Narratives, stories and anecdotes also play a role in the education of doctors; Macnaughton has argued that doctors learn primarily by the collection of stories about patients which can be referred to as 'illness scripts'.[37] It is thought that doctors on a subconscious level tend to compare the patient in front of them with a remembered illness script.[33] The continuing tradition of Balint groups also points out that story telling, and the reflective discussion in groups which case-based stories encourage, continue to be a valued form of professional development and education.

Finally, in research, narratives can set a patient-centred agenda, can challenge received wisdom and are potent agents in the generation of new research hypotheses. The use of patient narrative within the research account has the effect of keeping the uniqueness of individual encounter at the centre of practice, and in creating a body of stories about illness which can be used as a source of reflection on personal practice, for teaching and for developing studies which test out interventions at the level of patient, doctor or practice.

An example of the reflective use of narrative comes from recent research on asthma, which also explores the experiences of patients who may have a different language and culture to their doctor. This study by Griffiths and others used the narrative experience of patients to explore some of the dimensions of the doctor–patient relationship which contribute to high and low hospital admission rates. It appeared that admission rates were lower where patients had good access to doctors in practices with well-developed strategies to avoid admission, including a partnership style of consulting. Developing this style of relationship seemed more difficult for South Asian patients, who instead relied upon family advocacy to negotiate care and had less confidence in controlling their illness and initiating changes in medication.[38]

The future of relationship-based general practice

British general practice has been the envy of most of the Western world, with the registered list, longitudinal continuity of care and personal care being seen as the key structural elements which have contributed to its success.[39] Out of this reasonably stable structure has emerged a substantive body of theoretical and empirical work which has illuminated the nature of the doctor–patient relationship. An understanding of the behavioural elements of the consultation, alongside the diagnostic and therapeutic uses to which a reflective relationship can be put, has transformed the clinical teaching of general practice and influenced medical school teaching more generally.

It seems ironic that after 50 years in which these values have been extolled, and in which time there has been enormous change in the content of the job, we are entering a period when we are at risk of losing some of these things.

The context of the consultation and the doctor–patient relationship has changed in a number of significant ways, including an expanded professional agenda to encompass anticipatory and chronic care, and the expectation of a participatory consultation style. Longitudinal and personal continuity has become more difficult to maintain as practice teams get larger, and with increasing demand for part-time practice work from both women and men. Both patients and doctors have become part of a more mobile population.

Other changes in context are related to health service reforms which can be illustrated by conflicts over the time available for consultations. While it has been shown that extending the length of the consultation leads to better outcomes – including lower rates of prescribing, more health promotion activity, better recognition and management of psychosocial problems and better patient enablement – we are entering an era in which issues of access and choice have become a government priority.[29] The development of initiatives which bypass general practice, such as walk-in centres and NHS Direct, inevitably involves the reduplication of story telling and the potential for conflicting advice. Perversely these initiatives may work to erode patient trust and continuity, which are both aspects of personal care important for the management of chronic disease and minor illness which presents at the boundary between illness and disease.[40]

We may need to think afresh. Striking the right balance between access and continuity requires that we know which groups of patients both want and benefit from personal doctoring, and for which problems. We need to find out how to provide enabling personal care within communities where the doctor and patient may not share a common language, or a common stock of interpretations of illness presentations. The challenge must be to continue to work at expressing the components of personal care, the role of interpretation at the boundary between illness and disease, the role of advocate and of witness to the unfolding narrative of illness in a person's life. We need to maintain these core components during a time of substantial uncertainty as the shape of the new contract for general practice emerges.

Above all we need to assert that the relationship-based practice, expressed through consultations which are long enough to allow both for the increasing complexity of problems and for the participatory style of consultation which has been shown to be most effective and most valued by patients, remains at the core of general practice. We must ensure that these aspects of the discipline form an essential component of the quality criteria by which general practice in the future will be evaluated.

References

1   Foucault M (1973) *The Birth of the Clinic*. Tavistock Publications, London.

2   Balint M (1957) *The Doctor, His Patient and the Illness*. Tavistock Publications, London.

3   Morrell D (1998) As I recall. *BMJ*. **317**: 40–5.

4   Hull SA (1996) The method of Balint group work and its contribution to research in general practice. *Family Practice*. **13** (Suppl. 1): S10–2.

5   Balint M, Hunt J, Joyce D *et al.* (1970) *Treatment or Diagnosis: a study of repeat prescriptions in general practice*. Tavistock Publications, London.

6   Balint E and Norrell J (eds) (1973) *Six Minutes for the Patient: interactions in general practice consultations*. Tavistock Publications, London.

7   Balint E, Courtenay M, Elder A *et al.* (1993) *The Doctor, the Patient and the Group*. Routledge, London.

8   Harris C (1989) Seeing sunflowers: the William Pickles lecture. *Journal of the Royal College of General Practitioners*. **39**: 313–19.

9   Brown K and Freeling P (1976) *The Doctor–Patient Relationship*. Churchill Livingstone, Edinburgh.

10 Morrell DC (1981) *An Introduction to Primary Medical Care*. Churchill Livingstone, Edinburgh.

11 Tudor Hart J (1988) *A New Kind of Doctor*. Merlin Press, London.

12 Royal College of General Practitioners (1972) *The Future General Practitioner: learning and teaching*. RCGP, London.

13 www.Balint.co.uk The website of the Balint Society, which is dedicated to helping GPs towards a better understanding of the emotional content of the doctor–patient relationship.

14 Salinsky J and Sakin P (2000) *What are You Feeling, Doctor?* Radcliffe Medical Press, Oxford.

15 Gilley J (1988) Intimacy and terminal care. *Journal of the Royal College of General Practitioners.* **38**: 121–2.

16 Thomas KB (1987) General practice consultations: is there any point in being positive? *BMJ.* **294**: 1200–2.

17 Savage R and Armstrong D (1990) Effect of a GP's consulting style on patient's satisfaction: a controlled study. *BMJ.* **301**: 968–70.

18 Little P, Everitt H, Williamson I *et al.* (2001) Observational study of effect of patient-centredness and positive approach on outcomes of general practice consultations. *BMJ.* **323**: 908–11.

19 Pendleton D and Hasler J (eds) (1983) *Doctor–Patient Communication*. Academic Press, London.

20 Byrne PS and Long BEL (1976) *Doctors Talking to Patients*. HMSO, London.

21 Stott NCH and Davis RH (1979) The exceptional potential in each primary care consultation. *Journal of the Royal College of General Practitioners.* **29**: 201–5.

22 Kleinman A (1980) *Patients and Healers in the Context of Culture*. University of California Press, Berkeley.

23 Becker MH and Maiman LA (1975) Sociobehavioural determinants of compliance with health and medical care recommendations. *Medical Care.* **13**: 10–24.

24 Tuckett D, Boulton M, Olson C *et al.* (1985) *Meetings Between Experts*. Tavistock Publications, London.

25 Pendleton D, Schofield T, Tate P *et al.* (1984) *The Consultation: an approach to learning and teaching*. Oxford University Press, Oxford.

26 Freeman GK and Hjortdahl P (1997) What future for continuity of care in general practice? *BMJ.* **314**: 1870–80.

27 Williams SJ and Calnan M (1991) Key determinants of consumer satisfaction with general practice. *Family Practice.* **8**: 237–42.

28 Greenhalgh T (2002) Intuition and evidence – uneasy bedfellows. *British Journal of General Practice.* **52**: 395–400.

29 Howie JGR, Heaney DJ, Maxwell M *et al.* (1999) Quality at general practice consultations: cross-sectional survey. *BMJ.* **319**: 738–44.

30 Ettlinger P and Freeman G (1981) General practice compliance study: is it worth being a personal doctor? *BMJ.* **282**: 1192–4.

31 Kearley K, Freeman G and Heath A (2001) An exploration of the personal doctor–patient relationship in general practice. *British Journal of General Practice.* **51**: 712–18.

32 Marinker M (1998) The narrative of Hilda Thompson. In: Greenhalgh T and Hurwitz B (eds) *Narrative-based Medicine.* BMJ Books, London.

33 Greenhalgh T and Hurwitz B (eds) (1998) *Narrative-based Medicine.* BMJ Books, London.

34 Toon PD (1999) *Towards a Philosophy of General Practice: a study of the virtuous practitioner.* Royal College of General Practitioners, London.

35 Heath I (1995) *The Mystery of General Practice.* The Nuffield Provincial Hospitals Trust, London.

36 Holmes J (1998) Narrative in psychotherapy. In: Greenhalgh T and Hurwitz B (eds) *Narrative-based Medicine.* BMJ Books, London.

37 Macnaughton J (1998) Anecdote in clinical practice. In: Greenhalgh T and Hurwitz B (eds) *Narrative-based Medicine.* BMJ Books, London.

38 Griffiths C, Kaur G, Gantley M *et al.* (2001) Influences on hospital admission for asthma in South Asian and white adults: qualitative interview study. *BMJ.* **323**: 962.

39 Hjordahl P (2001) Continuity of care – going out of style? *British Journal of General Practice.* **51**: 699–700.

40 Freeman GK, Horder J, Howie JGR *et al.* (2002) Evolving general practice consultation in Britain: issues of length and context. *BMJ.* **324**: 880–2.

CHAPTER 8

Fifty years of research in general practice

Yvonne H Carter and Amanda Howe

The importance of research in primary healthcare

General practice and primary care are at the heart of decision making in the National Health Service (NHS). Effective and efficient primary healthcare is characterised by its accessibility as 'first point of contact', its longitudinal relationship with patients, its focus on the person as well as their illnesses, its responsibility for dealing with the most common problems in the population, its coordinating function for integrated patient care and its orientation to prevention and population health in addition to traditional clinical functions.[1,2] As an academic discipline, general practice has achieved a remarkable position in the international healthcare scene during the past 50 years. In the UK, over 90% of contacts between the population and the NHS take place in primary care and over recent years there has been a shift in care from the hospital to the community. The opportunities for research are great, but as a field of research it is still relatively underexplored and the evidence base for primary care needs to be strengthened. This chapter explores the importance of research in primary healthcare, the key historical milestones and recent organisational developments, including capacity and capability building for research in general practice teams and new primary care organisations.

A balanced portfolio of research in and on primary care is essential if the discipline is to progress at both clinical and organisational levels. All members of the primary healthcare team need a range of information to support their decisions. Research *in* primary care provides the clinical generalist with the means to test and improve clinical practice, evaluate innovative models of service delivery and to understand population data. Research *on* primary care provides the means to improve organisation of services and to question local beliefs or behaviours on the basis of population data. Much of the evidence base required by primary care can *only* be obtained by research and development (R&D) in primary care that involves primary care practitioners and their patients.[3] A multidisciplinary approach is required in health services, public health and primary care research to address the broad range of objectives identified within areas for future research as exemplified by recent priority-setting exercises[4-6] in the UK. The appropriate involvement of primary care staff in research is also likely to increase the quality of clinical care in the NHS. Primary care organisations have a vital role to play in the development of a research culture.

History and key milestones

Founded in 1952, the College of General Practitioners concentrated on research, immediately and instinctively recognising it as a main challenge.[7] Officers at that time recognised three key obstacles: professional isolation, lack of skills and experience in research, and a failure of general practice to penetrate the universities. The Research Committee was one of only four committees formed in 1953. Despite the lack of resources and tradition, all five members held a Doctorate in Medicine. There was a clear intent to promote quality and high standards. The research newsletter, a research register and the first steps towards a national morbidity survey quickly followed.

Pickles, the first president of the RCGP, demonstrated that world-class research could be done by GPs working entirely outside of the hospital environment.[7] He traced the spread of some infectious diseases within his practice population and threw new light on the period of their infectivity. Fry, another early research pioneer, highlighted the important role of family doctors in the continuity of care of patients. He achieved much from within the confines of a single general practice and did a great deal to make research in the setting of ordinary everyday practice a reality. He is particularly known for describing the profiles of disease.[8] His description of GP researchers still holds true today: those working alone, those working with others, those gathering information from others and those willing to develop and test research methods in their own practices. In other words, these are the 'investigators and collaborators' we now regularly refer to within primary care teams.

The RCGP currently has two Research Units, whose Directors report to the College's Council through the Chairman of Research.[7,9] The Birmingham Unit, established by Crombie, and now led by Fleming, is older than any university department of general practice. It is perhaps best known for its successful role in the national morbidity surveys and the weekly returns service from the sentinel practices. The Manchester Unit, initially under the leadership of Kay, exploited the developing research interest in contraception and especially the oral contraceptive pill. This has resulted in the largest collective research study ever undertaken in the world with GP records. In 1997, the Unit relocated to the University of Aberdeen where it is currently known as the RCGP Centre for Primary Care Research and Epidemiology.

Before the 1950s there were no primary care lecturers on the staff of universities, nor a single Chair of General Practice in a university department anywhere in the world. There were precious few role models to inspire or encourage the new generation of GP researchers. The first independent University Department of General Practice and first Chair of General Practice were established in Edinburgh in 1957 and 1963 respectively. The recipient, Scott, had previously been appointed to the staff of the University of Edinburgh in 1956 through the support of social medicine (public health). Other medical schools were slow to follow Edinburgh's lead: Byrne was not appointed to the first Chair in England at Manchester until 1972. Each of the undergraduate medical schools in the UK now has an academic Department and Professor of General Practice/Primary Care and this pattern has continued around the world, showing that general practice can be more than simply a teaching facility for a medical school.

The development of general practice as a university discipline has been reviewed by Harris in 1969,[10] Byrne in 1973[11] and in the Mackenzie Report in 1986.[12] The reviews led to a number of organisational reforms in the UK. Although the pace of development of university departments of general practice or family medicine has been reasonably good internationally in terms of entry to a large number of institutions in a relatively short time, the infrastructure support for them has often been unsatisfactory with shortage of accommodation, support staff and lack of tenured posts. Initially the trend was to appoint single individuals or small groups. More recently the general pattern has been to blur the boundaries between departments and grow into large interdisciplinary teams working with colleagues across community health sciences. Working in partnership with networks of teaching and research-active practices, a multiprofessional approach is illustrated by the variety of disciplines currently working within academic departments of general practice/primary care. These may include doctors, nurses, managers, social scientists, anthropologists, statisticians, psychologists and others.

In 1999, Wallace delivered a keynote address on the momentum to develop the academic agenda in family medicine in Europe, and examined mechanisms to promote linkage between clinical work, research and education.[13] However, the progress towards an established career structure within academic general practice has been slow. In 2002 the Heads of Departments from the Society of Academic Primary Care (previously the Association of University Departments of General Practice) analysed a survey of the current composition and key activities across research and undergraduate and postgraduate education, and the clinical effectiveness of UK departments. The preliminary findings suggest that the increased capacity has not yet stabilised within the higher education setting, and this poses a threat to the fulfilment of the 'joined-up thinking' in Wallace's address.

The development of research practices and networks

During the 1990s, the Department of Health and the Medical Research Council gave increased recognition to research in primary care.[3-6,14,15] In the UK, many primary care organisations are now more actively involved in research; this includes academic departments of general practice and primary care, and other university departments engaged in health services research or social science, cooperatives of individual practices and the primary care research networks (PCRNs). Gray *et al.*[16] attempted to map the extent of involvement of 1031 general practices in the south and west regions of England in undergraduate medical school teaching, medical vocational training, continuing medical education and research. More than half the practices were actively involved in either teaching or research, with 15% involved in both. It is interesting to note that all practices with a leading role in research were also involved in teaching.

Kernick *et al.*[17] have identified research practices as key to development and to sustaining change. The first 'dedicated' research practice in the UK was appointed by the RCGP in 1994 and provided with limited financial support to cover infrastructure costs. Since this time the scheme has been evaluated,[18] and there have been similar developments through regional and national research and development offices.[19,20] The development of research practices allows individual primary care teams to become more involved in research at a variety of levels. They may be involved in community-based pharmaceutical trials or be working in collaboration with local university departments or with acute or community hospitals.

In 1998, the RCGP developed a pilot scheme to accredit UK general practices undertaking primary care research and development. The Assessment Schedule included two levels: a Collaborative Research Practice with little direct experience of gaining project or infrastructure funding; or an Established Research Practice with more experience of research funding and activity and a sound infrastructure to allow for growth in capacity. The process for assessment involved the review of written documentation and an assessment visit by a multidisciplinary team. In 2001, recommendations were made to formally launch the scheme, renamed Primary Care Research Team Assessment (PCRTA). The role of primary care research networks has been highlighted in relation to support and mentoring for research practices undergoing assessment. The new assessment scheme will help primary care trusts and individual practices to prepare and demonstrate their approach to research governance in a systematic way.[21]

Inspired by the early surveillance systems in the UK and the Netherlands, PCRNs have been established internationally to develop research and education in primary healthcare and implement research evidence.[22] Networks as virtual organisations use different organisational approaches to enable multidisciplinary coalitions of researchers, promote ownership of research activity and disseminate information efficiently. The last 20 years has seen the further enhancement of the Medical Research Council's General Practice Research Framework in the UK with a membership of over 1000 practices.[23] Networks have developed rapidly across many countries, mirroring changes in funding and research infrastructure. They are diverse in their aims, governance, size, organisational structure, methods of delivery, research interests and training needs of their members.[24–32] They generally reflect a need to strengthen and develop the research base of primary care. In 1998, Fleming proposed a helpful theoretical classification to describe the functions of research networks (*see* Box 8.1).[33]

Primary care research networks have been characterised as either 'top down' or 'bottom up' according to whether their primary purpose is to meet commissioners' or members' needs respectively.[34] Whatever their approach, the emergence and success of networks in recent years has provided an important infrastructure for primary care research. Networks have made a great deal of progress in relation to research methods training and have begun to contribute important information to the primary care knowledge base. The growth and facilitatory role of networks in relation to primary care mean that they may have an important role to play in relation to the development, support and assessment of research practices. The Federation of Primary Care Research Networks has provided a useful umbrella organisation to represent the views and organisational needs of its members.[35]

Box 8.1   Functions of networks

Networks providing epidemiological data
- Sentinel networks providing early identification of health problems of public health importance
- Networks for morbidity surveys examining the patterns of diseases presented to healthcare
- Networks involved in both sentinel surveillance and epidemiological surveys providing evidence of diagnostic validation

Networks concerned with the process of care
- Quality assurance networks using methods such as review of prescribing patterns or audit against predetermined standards
- Focused networks dealing with a particular problem
- Networks for clinical trials

There is no doubt that PCRNs have provided an important infrastructure for primary care research and there is a growing body of literature that confirms that networks are feasible and capable of important research. Networks have contributed to capacity building, facilitating collaborative research partnerships and providing access to methodological support and training. Little evaluative work, however, has been undertaken on the role and structure of networks themselves on a national or international scale.[24] Questions remain about the role that PCRNs play in enhancing research activity, promoting evidence-based healthcare and providing better 'value for money' than alternative strategies for developing R&D in primary care.

Contribution to clinical standards and evidence-based primary healthcare

In the UK in recent years the National Institute for Clinical Excellence (NICE) has had an important role in providing the NHS with consistent and timely guidance on what is best for patients.[36,37] NICE has advised on the value of clinical interventions across the health service and also provided guidelines and clinical audit packages. General practice, however, has been a useful experimental field for implementation research; for example, the early work on guideline development demonstrated how little effect passive dissemination has on professional practice.[38] Many questions about guidelines implementation remain: how can we implement more than one guideline at a time, particularly in a time of rapidly expanding numbers of National Service Frameworks? Are nurse educators as effective as doctors in changing practice? How can we prolong the effect of an intervention? How can we implement multi-agency guidelines across primary and secondary care and across a primary care group/trust?[39]

Primary care is now a substantial presence in domains of clinical research which were previously the preserve of secondary care academics. Evidence from primary care studies is routinely included in systematic reviews informing NICE and other clinical guidelines. Primary care researchers are also gaining skills and expertise in designing randomised trials and conducting reviews and meta-analyses.[40–45] Researchers in primary care have carried out studies on different clinical topics, adapting methods from various disciplines to assess the impact that clinical guidelines have on the quality of individual patient care.[46,47]

Many methodological challenges remain: for example, outcomes that are commonly used to assess effectiveness of the health service (death, disability, hospitalisation) are relatively uncommon in primary care, even in high-risk groups. Studies which use these to assess the effect of an intervention are generally too large for a local – and sometimes national – study. In primary care research it is often necessary to use process measures signifying quality of care (e.g. appropriate prescribing) or intermediate outcomes (e.g. patient symptoms). In spite of the maturation of general practice as an academic discipline, its diversity remains, and thus many different methods and approaches may be valuable in illuminating different research questions. Unfortunately, not all such research is equally desirable to funders, and this can compound some of the contemporary challenges outlined below.

Capacity and capability for research

Over the last decade GPs and their attached staff have been increasingly recognised as being in an ideal position to address the health needs of their patients, to create a critical mass of research activity and to bid for specific funding for primary care-based research. However, training for family doctors and primary and community nurses has historically provided little experience in research methods. Lack of protected time, resources and infrastructure have been persistent barriers to progression.

In 1997, the *Report of an Independent Task Force on Clinical Academic Careers*[48] in the UK reported that almost every medical school had difficulty in recruiting academic staff in general practice. The report acknowledged that some significant improvements in the overall conditions of service for GP academics would be needed for the discipline to prosper. The last few years has seen a flurry of policy publications relevant to the further development of the discipline.[3–6,14,15] The reports identified an urgent need to expand the research capacity in primary care from its historical low base, where research was poorly funded yet fundamental to raising the quality of patient care. Recommendations include the need to: increase the recruitment, development and retention of R&D leaders in primary care; increase the number of clinical staff with R&D expertise; increase the involvement of staff in non-clinical disciplines and achieve an evidence-based culture in primary care. Following publication of the report *R&D in Primary Care*,[3] the NHS R&D Programme launched the National Primary Care Awards Scheme. The scheme is intended to identify in national competition individuals of the highest calibre who wish to pursue a career in health-related primary care research. The scheme seeks to 'fast-track' such individuals by supporting them in a customised research training environment that reflects their individual talents and training needs.

Many academic departments now provide teaching on research methods with an increasing number of diploma courses, masters degrees and PhD studentships being developed for postgraduate students.[49] Courses have been responsive to the changing needs of primary care and aim to offer modularity with improved accessibility and a menu to allow personal development in teaching, research and a range of contemporary issues. These are clearly to be welcomed in higher professional training for GPs and other primary care staff.

New posts are being created for GP registrars and young family doctors with protected time for personal development and research. There can be tensions in balancing different academic responsibilities with clinical work and personal learning needs.[50] Flexible posts with linked clinical and protected academic sessions can aid recruitment and retention of GPs in inner-city practices. These posts may be linked to a taught masters programme in research methods.

Young primary care practitioners are particularly expecting flexibility with a choice of entry routes into academia and established career pathways. A number of opportunities exist which enable junior academics to develop their research skills under the personal supervision of a senior academic, whilst undertaking a research project related to general practice.[51–53] Across Europe, a research doctorate (MD or PhD) is a prerequisite for an academic career leading to a professorship of general practice.[54] This can be interpreted as strengthening the academic base of primary healthcare.

Status of primary healthcare research in the NHS

A key challenge for university-based departments is the decision either to stay focused on clinical general practice or to develop wider expertise in health service research. The quality of the research versus teaching load also needs to be carefully considered. Will there only be a few research-based departments and will they have to have a full quota of expertise in qualitative epidemiology, economics and statistics to be successful in gaining grants from the prestigious research charities? Arguments of critical mass come into play here. Does this mean integrating primary care research with health services research and public health? This is becoming a global problem. The tension here is between research that is generalisable and of international stature and the development of a wider base of research-ready clinicians.

The next major challenge involves links to the new primary care organisation. What is the future for PCRNs? Are they really about high-quality research that is generalisable? Or are they awareness-raising and capacity-building networks? The same problem applies to research practices – what are their aims? The increasing in-roads made by commercial/pharmaceutical companies into clinical trials in primary care are an added complicating factor.

Opportunities to engage in R&D in primary care are growing and the scope for those wishing to become involved is finally widening. Infrastructure funding for research-active practices and the evolution of PCRNs have helped to improve the research capacity and blur some of the boundaries between academic departments and clinical practice. We are beginning to see an increase in primary care-based research, which is in turn leading to an increase in an evidence base for decision making by GPs and other disciplines working in primary care. The role of primary care trusts (PCTs) in relation to primary care research is still unclear. Teaching PCTs are already developing and the evolution of research PCTs is about to blossom. Research-active PCTs with leadership for research governance and management across a geographical area may emerge from a research practice or individual, others from existing networks or links with university departments or R&D units.[55,56]

What is the role of the RCGP in securing a future for primary care research?

The importance of research was recognised by the College's founders. The preceding sections set out a rich history of research enthusiasm and productivity that spans the evidence base of daily practice, the novice or 'dabbler' enjoying a research methods course and the cutting-edge research that embraces both academics and clinicians, patients and professors. While the College's mission is not solely academic (though indeed it is sometimes falsely accused of being 'for academics'!), the recognition of the value and necessity of research to excellence in primary care has made its role in the College increasingly visible over the first half century. The College has supported research through its Scientific Foundation Board and Fellowships; run training events and produced publications, such as the Research Master Class Series; recognised achievement through awards such as the RCGP/Boots Research Paper of the Year; and continues to lobby actively to secure and enhance NHS R&D funding opportunities across the UK. Key roles for the RCGP over the next 50 years are to ensure that: basic research skills become a core competence of every GP, and indeed of most members of the primary care team; practices increasingly seek to host research and contribute to the growing sophistication of the evidence base of the discipline; it champions research-based career opportunities, alongside the portfolio of clinical, political and educational special interests; and it bridges the divide between universities and the service through effective structural links and partnerships. The gains for patients, staff, learners and other clinical disciplines will be invaluable.

References

1   Royal College of General Practitioners (1996) *The Nature of General Medical Practice.* Occasional Paper 27. RCGP, London.

2   Starfield B (1994) Is primary care essential? *Lancet.* **344**: 1129–33.

3   Mant D (1997) *National Working Group on R&D in Primary Care: final report.* NHS Executive, London.

4 Medical Research Council (1997) *Primary Health Care* [topic review]. MRC, London.

5 Department of Health (2000) *Research and Development for a First Class Service: R&D funding in the new NHS.* DoH, Leeds.

6 Department of Health (2000) *NHS R&D Funding. Consultation Paper: NHS priorities and needs funding.* DoH, Leeds.

7 Royal College of General Practitioners (1992) *Forty Years On. The Story of the First Forty Years of the Royal College of General Practitioners.* RCGP, London.

8 Fry J (1966) *Profiles of Disease. A Study in the Natural History of Common Diseases.* E & S Livingstone, Edinburgh.

9 Carter YH, Elwyn G and Hungin P (2001) *General Practitioner Research at the Millennium. A Perspective from the RCGP.* Royal College of General Practitioners, London.

10 Harris CM (1969) *General Practice Teaching of Undergraduates in British Medical Schools.* Reports from General Practice No. XI. Royal College of General Practitioners, London.

11 Byrne PS (1973) University departments of general practice and the undergraduate teaching of general practice in the United Kingdom in 1972. *Journal of the Royal College of General Practitioners.* **23** (1): 1–12.

12 Howie JGR, Hannay DR and Stevenson JSK (1986) *The Mackenzie Report: general practice in the medical schools of the United Kingdom, 1986.* University of Edinburgh, Edinburgh.

13 Wallace P (1999) Building bridges: integrating research and undergraduate education into general practice/family medicine. *European Journal of General Practice.* **5**: 116–19.

14 Research and Development Task Force (1994) *Supporting Research and Development in the NHS.* A report to the Minister for Health by a Research and Development Task Force chaired by Professor Anthony Culyer. HMSO, London.

15 NHS Executive (1998) *Developing Human Resources for Health-related R&D: next steps.* Report of the R&D Workforce Capacity Development Group. Department of Health, London.

16 Gray S, Toth B, Johnson H *et al.* (2000) Mapping teaching and research activity in general practice. *Medical Teacher.* **22**: 64–9.

17 Kernick D, Stead J and Dixon M (1999) Moving the research agenda to where it matters. *BMJ.* **319**: 206–7.

18 Sibbald B and Dowell J (1998) *RCGP Research Practices: an evaluation.* National Primary Care Research and Development Centre, Manchester.

19 Smith LFP (1997) Research general practices: what, who and why? *British Journal of General Practice.* **47**: 83–6.

20 Wright D and Smith H (1999) *Evaluation of Designated Research Practices: interim report.* Wessex Primary Care Research Network, Southampton.

21 Carter YH, Shaw S and Macfarlane F (2002) *Primary Care Research Team Assessment (PCRTA): development and evaluation.* Occasional Paper 81. Royal College of General Practitioners, London.

22 Green LA and Dovey SA (2001) Practice-based primary care research networks. *BMJ.* **322**: 567–8.

23 Vickers M, Hand L and Hand C (1999) The MRC General Practice Research Framework. In: Carter Y and Thomas C (eds) *Research Opportunities in Primary Care.* Radcliffe Medical Press, Oxford.

24 Carter YH, Shaw S and Sibbald B (2000) Primary care research networks: an evolving model meriting national evaluation. *British Journal of General Practice.* **460**: 859–60.

25 Hungin P and Rubin G (2001) Are primary care research networks up to the challenge? *Primary Health Care Research and Development.* **2**: 67–8.

26 Thomas P, Kai J, O'Dwyer A *et al.* (2000) Primary care groups and research networks: opportunities for R&D in context. *British Journal of General Practice.* **50**: 91–2.

27 Griffiths F, Wild A, Harvey J *et al.* (2000) The productivity of primary care research networks. *British Journal of General Practice.* **50**: 913–15.

28 Evans D, Exworthy M, Peckham S *et al.* (1997) *Primary Care Research Networks: report to the NHS Executive South and West Research and Development Directorate.* Institute for Health Policy Studies, University of Southampton.

29 Hungin P, Kendrick T, Moore M *et al.* (1999) Research networks. In: Carter Y and Thomas K (eds) *Research Opportunities in Primary Care.* Radcliffe Medical Press, Oxford.

30 Nutting P (1996) Practice-based research networks: building the infrastructure of primary care research. *Journal of Family Practice.* **42** (2): 199–203.

31 Rait G, Rogers S and Wallace P (2002) Primary care research networks: perspectives, research interests and training needs of its members. *Primary Health Care Research and Development.* **3**: 4–10.

32 Thomas P (2001) Next steps for primary care research networks. *Primary Health Care Research and Development.* **2**: 137–8.

33 Fleming DM (1998) The role of research networks in primary care. *European Journal of General Practice.* **4**: 96–9.

34 Thomas P, Griffiths F, Kai J *et al.* (2001) Networks for research in primary health care. *BMJ.* **322**: 588–90.

35 Smith H (2000) The Federation of Primary Care Research Networks: a national initiative to enhance networking locally. *Primary Health Care Research and Development.* **1**: 3–4.

36 Dent THS and Sadler M (2002) From guidance to practice: why NICE is not enough. *BMJ.* **324**: 842–5.

37 Sculper M, Drummond M and O'Brien B (2001) Effectiveness, efficiency and NICE. *BMJ.* **322**: 943–4.

38 Grimshaw JM and Russell IT (1993) Effect of clinical guidelines on medical practice: a systematic review of rigorous evaluations. *Lancet.* **342**: 1317–22.

39 Feder G, Cryer C, Donovan S *et al.* (2000) Guidelines for the prevention of falls in older people. *BMJ.* **321**: 1007–11.

40 Bower P, Byford S, Sibbald B *et al.* (2000) Randomised controlled trial of non-directive counselling, cognitive behaviour therapy, and usual general practitioner care for patients with depression. *BMJ.* **321**: 1389–92.

41 Little P, Williamson I, Warner G *et al.* (1997) An open randomised trial of prescribing strategies for sore throat. *BMJ.* **314**: 722–7.

42 Kinmonth A, Woodcock A, Griffin S *et al.* Randomised controlled trial of patient-centred care of diabetes in general practice: impact on current well-being and future disease risk. *BMJ.* **317**: 1202–8.

43 Horrocks S, Anderson E and Salisbury C (2002) Systematic review of whether nurse practitioners working in primary care can provide equivalent care to doctors. *BMJ.* **324**: 819–23.

44 Silagy C, Mant D, Fowler G *et al.* (1994) Meta-analysis of efficacy of nicotine replacement therapies in smoking cessation. *Lancet.* **343**: 139–42.

45 Schroeder K and Fahey T (2002) Systematic review of randomised controlled trials of over-the-counter cough medicines for acute cough in adults. *BMJ.* **324**: 329–31.

46 Feder G, Griffiths C, Spence M *et al.* (1996) Do guidelines-derived postal prompts to survivors of myocardial infarction or unstable angina and to their GPs improve secondary prevention? *Family Practice.* **13**: 346.

47 Feder G, Griffiths C, Highton C *et al.* (1995) Do clinical guidelines introduced with practice-based education improve care of asthmatic and diabetic patients? *BMJ.* **311**: 1473–8.

48 Committee of Vice Chancellors and Principals (1997) *Clinical Academic Careers: Report of an Independent Task Force.* CVCP, London.

49 Hilton S and Carter YH (2000) Academic careers in general practice and primary care. *Medical Education.* **34**: 910–15.

50 Lester HE, Carter YH, Dawood D *et al.* (1998) Survey of research activity, training needs, departmental support and career intentions of junior academic general practitioners. *British Journal of General Practice.* **48**: 1322–6.

51 Rosser W (2001) Academic careers in primary care. *Medical Education.* **35**: 99.

52 Carter YH and Green F (2000) An academic career. In: Baker M and Chambers R (eds) *The Great Careers Debate in General Practice.* Royal College of General Practitioners, London.

53 Howe A, Carter YH, Thomas K *et al.* (2000) *Undertaking Higher Degrees: some practical guidance.* Royal College of General Practitioners, London.

54 Kochen MM and Himmel W (2000) Academic careers in general practice: scientific requirements in Europe. *European Journal of General Practice.* **6**: 62–7.

55 Kernick D, Stead J and Carter YH (2002) Developing primary care research: primary care trusts – a natural home? *Primary Health Care Research and Development.* **3**: 71–3.

56 Jones R, Carter YH and Hilton S (2002) New arrangements for NHS R&D funding: implications for primary care research. *British Journal of General Practice.* **52**: 7–8.

CHAPTER 9

The general practitioner as a teacher

Amanda Howe and Yvonne H Carter

Introduction

There is a saying that 'a bad GP teaches no one anything, but a good GP can always teach anyone something'. The two authors of this chapter are agreed that as we have become older, we are ever less inclined to see anyone as wholly 'good' or 'bad', especially when we see how much performance is influenced by circumstances. Nevertheless, there is good evidence that GPs are often also good teachers, as we have witnessed repeatedly in our professional lifetimes. This chapter looks at the 'who, what and why' of GPs as teachers, and suggests that this under-acknowledged component of our discipline's practice should be embraced as part of our core task in the future.

A moment on definitions

First, a definition: 'teacher' and 'teaching' in this chapter denote the role played by a GP when consciously attempting to assist someone else to gain under-standing which may be important to their current or future role. This therefore includes the frequent role of 'teacher' within the consultation, but does not include unconscious behaviours – from which others may nevertheless draw important conclusions. For example, as a child we learned 'how you should behave when with a doctor' without the doctor having to teach us that as such (the doctor's actions, aided and abetted by repeated maternal instruc-tions before – and reward or punishment afterwards – did the trick). Similarly, a medical student may base their behaviour towards colleagues on their obser-vations of how other doctors treat team members over time. Such behaviours may therefore be a source of learning: the skill of a teacher comes into play when an effort is made to assist the learner to bring such unconscious knowledge into the conscious domain – in order to reflect on it, critique it and make it useful.

Second, why 'teaching' rather than 'learning'? In these days of self-directed learning, teaching has an unfashionably didactic tone: this is not the intention for this chapter, where the term implies the role that the GP voluntarily plays in the learning process. The learner is the one who does the learning, while the GP assists them by acting in a teaching capacity (which could include sitting in silence if this is the most effective method).

What teaching do GPs do?

The changing role of medicine in society and the growing expectations that patients have of their doctors mean that the content and delivery of medical curricula have had to change over recent years.[1] There has been a shift in the focus of healthcare from episodic care of individual patients in hospitals to the promotion of health in the community. This has been accompanied by a change in approach from paternalism and anecdotal care to seeing the patient as an equal partner, in a negotiated management based on evidence of clinical effectiveness and safety, and informed by personal preference. Medical training has become more student-centred, with an emphasis on active learning rather than on the passive acquisition of knowledge, and on the assessment of clinical competence rather than on the ability to retain and recall unrelated facts.[2]

So what do GPs teach? With a *patient or carer*, they are likely to be teaching about the nature of an illness and how it can be investigated and treated. They may also be teaching about agencies and technical aids that can help the patient with their problem. Sometimes, they are teaching from their professional experience of life; for example, doctors often know much more about the experience of bereavement than their patients since it is a frequent event in general practice. In most consultations they will also be addressing self-care and ways in which the patient can make best use of the services available.

With *'official learners'* (for example, medical students or GP registrars), they will be teaching to a wide variety of learning objectives. Some examples of specific curricula will be given later, but the aim of a teaching session could range from a practical skill (writing a prescription for a controlled drug) to complex psycho-dynamic issues (how to use empathy as a psychological tool to reduce potential dependency in the doctor–patient relationship).

With *colleagues*, they are more likely to be co-learning; for example, a GP and nurse may agree to run a shared triage clinic for urgent access requests and will need to learn from each other which tasks are best suited to their different competencies. In this example, however, the GP will certainly be 'teaching' to some extent as the nurse is taking on a task which the GP can already perform. Thus another criterion of teaching emerges: if the GP has competencies needed but not yet held by the learner, the GP acts as teacher when assisting the other to acquire these competencies, even if the GP is also learning something new in the process. GPs often also teach colleagues outside their own practice because they have some expertise which is specifically valued: one example would be the role of GPs who share their research skills with other practices through organising collaborative research studies, or undertaking academic supervision of those doing higher degrees such as PhDs.[3]

Who do GPs teach?

The three core groups of *patients, those in training* and *colleagues*, are reasonably comprehensive categories. In most circumstances, it is those in training who are considered as formally 'taught' by the GP since they are in contact with the GP for the specific purpose of learning, rather than because they share a working environment or have a clinical need. GPs have taken on roles at all levels of medical education: as teachers for medical undergraduates in basic training, as specialist trainers of future GPs and as tutors to assist their peers in their continuing professional development.[4] Many GPs contribute to the training of other disciplines; for example, paramedics or nurses. There is also an increasing number of GPs whose key educational role is to 'teach the teachers' through their roles in universities and deaneries. For some GPs engaged in key strategic roles such as professorial posts or deans/directors of general practice, their teaching role is threefold: not only front-line teaching, but committed to developing the competencies of more junior members of their team, and teaching the nature and opportunities of primary care to other members of their institution.

One of the great pleasures of working in a multidisciplinary environment is the contribution made by different cultures, and both the health service and higher education institutions can usefully learn from the disciplines which coexist within them. Although the latter 'teaching' function may be opaque to some service practitioners, academic general practitioners play an important role in educating others about modern primary care and championing its capabilities against some outdated stereotypes (and the occasional clear-cut prejudice!). Without the historical 'champion' role of the RCGP and the associated national GP leaders, the opportunities for GPs to teach would be much curtailed; for example, there was only one UK medical school with a Professor of General Practice in 1962, but by 1972 11 out of 29 schools had GP input, and by the 50th year of the RCGP all new medical schools had a substantive GP role built into their core structure (of which more later).

Although there has been a tradition of teaching medical students in the setting of general practice, which dates back more than 200 years, there were no primary care lecturers on the staff of universities before the 1950s, nor a single Chair of General Practice in a university department anywhere in the world.

There were therefore precious few role models to inspire a new generation of researchers in primary care. The first independent University Department of General Practice and first Chair of General Practice were established in Edinburgh in 1957 and 1963 respectively. Other medical schools were slow to follow Edinburgh's lead. When the Dutch College of General Practitioners was formed in 1956, one of the aims was to promote a more general practice-oriented medical education. The consequence of the introduction of vocational training for GPs was that between 1966 and 1970 each Dutch Medical Faculty founded a Chair in General Practice. The departments of general practice were by origin very strongly education oriented.[5] Byrne was not appointed to the first Chair in England at Manchester until 1972 and the 1970s then saw a gradual acceleration of this process.

The development of general practice as a university discipline has been reviewed by Harris in 1969,[6] Byrne in 1973[7] and in the Mackenzie Report in 1986.[8] The reviews led to a number of organisational reforms in the UK. Although the pace of development of university departments of general practice or family medicine has been reasonable, the support for them has often been unsatisfactory as exemplified by shortages of accommodation, support personnel and the lack of tenured posts for academic staff. Initially the trend was to appoint single individuals or small groups. More recently the general pattern has been to grow into large interdisciplinary teams working with colleagues across community health sciences in partnership with networks of teaching and research-active practices. Senior appointments are being differentiated increasingly into either research or educational positions.

Why do GPs teach?

In yet another year of change and pressure and demand on primary care, it is interesting to ask this question. When asked in a survey and interview study,[9] GPs cited a variety of factors which had motivated them to undertake their role as teachers, summarised in Box 9.1 as the 'seven Rs'. These were then sustained by a combination of a 'cycle of satisfaction' (a 'feel-good' factor created by enjoyment, seeing learners progress and positive feedback); peer support from others playing the same role or supporting them in it and routinisation of the role into their professional routine. A recent survey[10] of the primary care community around a new medical school showed a surprising level of positive response in spite of an exceptionally intensive expectation of GP input, with 56% (80) of GP respondents in Norfolk and Suffolk expressing a definite interest in teaching medical students, 28% (40) expressing a possible interest and only 16% (22) no interest. The barriers cited were almost entirely related to personnel capacity in the face of high student numbers, lack of replacement workforce and practical concerns about physical capacity to host students.

> **Box 9.1**   The seven Rs that motivate GPs to undertake community-based teaching
>
> - **R**efreshment of knowledge and skills – helps my own knowledge base
> - **R**ecruitment and retention – brings people into the job
> - **R**esources – attracts additional resources
> - **R**evalidation – helps me with my CPD and revalidation
> - **R**eciprocity – someone taught me, I should teach too
> - **R**esponsibility – it's part of our professional role
> - **R**espect for professional status – learners respect teachers and their discipline

Financial resources seemed to be less relevant to motivation, varying according to the particular demand made on the GP and practice, and the attitude of the particular team or GP. A cross-sectional survey reported in 2001[11] that practice involvement in undergraduate education in east London was associated with higher scores on a range of organisational and performance quality indicators. The lower patient-related income of teaching practices was associated with smaller list sizes, and may only have been partially replaced by teaching income. Lower vacancy rates suggested that teaching practices were more attractive to doctors seeking partnership in east London, a largely deprived urban area. However, the sustainability of the situation cannot be guaranteed as long as education is not part of the core contractual commitment of GPs, as it remains a 'voluntary' activity.

Where do GPs teach?

While the obvious answer is 'in their practice', this is by no means the whole story. Box 9.2 summarises the many microsettings in which GPs are known to teach, and outlines the types of activity they may be supervising. There are some boundary issues here: 'on the job' teaching can occur in any work setting, but many of the formal opportunities outlined require additional space for supervision of the learner(s). As the educational role becomes more formal, so many practices and PCTs are beginning to perceive the need for physical infrastructure to be available for educational and training use on an ongoing basis. In the 1990s, many political battles were fought to try to secure monies for GPs to parallel those historically afforded to other NHS providers of education under the SIFT (Service Increment for Teaching) arrangements. It remains the case that most GPs teach in their own premises with minimal reimbursement, though this picture may change as larger, locally owned premises such as intermediate care facilities and PCT educational facilities are developed.

Box 9.2 Settings for GP teaching

In the practice
- In their own consultations
- Observing others consult (including indirect observation, e.g. video)
- In the community context (home visits, health needs assessments)

- Demonstration of specific techniques (clinical skills, practical procedures)
- Tutorials

- Team learning sessions
- Audit and research projects

- Supervising student contacts and learning through patient follow-up projects

Outside the practice
- Lecturing and talks
- Group work with VT schemes or undergraduates

- Clinical and communication skills in hospital and/or university setting
- Teaching monitoring and accreditation (practice visits, peer review)
- Continuing medical education/continuing professional development posts
- Examining and assessment
- Teaching in other work-related settings (e.g. occupational health work, co-ops)
- Educational development (trainers, PCTs, university)

What do GPs need to be able to teach?

In recent years there has been an emphasis on providing quality undergraduate and postgraduate medical education that has focused attention on the educational responsibilities of all doctors. There has been a growing awareness of the need to train doctors as educators and a move towards an outcome-based approach in which competence in teaching is defined in a framework that supports the role of the teacher and encourages professionalism of teaching.[12]

If GPs are asked what they need to be able to teach, *time* is the usual answer volunteered. Many educational roles are very time consuming: for example, to be an MRCGP examiner is an onerous task that easily equates to the notional 30 hours per annum of expected continuing professional development. Some of the roles outlined necessitate the absence of the GP from the practice, or their dedicated time for supervision of the learner. The RCGP has argued strongly for recognition of such professional commitments in the GP 'portfolio' career structure, which in 2003 means that most GPs will wish to play a number of substantive roles outside their front-line service to patients during their working life. Educational commitments are only one subgroup of these roles, which may also include special clinical interests, PCT management roles and research activity.

GPs also need the *help of others* for successful fulfilment of their teaching roles. In most clinical settings the role of *the patient and their family* is central to learning: health students and trainees are absolutely reliant on the cooperation of the public to tell their stories, through which they learn the histories and symptoms of different clinical conditions. Contact with common and chronic illnesses is one of the great strengths which GP-based teaching brings to basic medical education; another is the opportunity to follow patients through cycles of life events, learn how they cope and understand the ways in which health professionals can help (or hinder) their progress. Similarly, GPs may need help from *other members of staff* and community-based agencies to fulfil some learning objectives, especially when demonstrating care pathways and use of team skills. Learners are more likely to thrive in a positive atmosphere, and the enthusiasm and help of the team is invaluable to the GP teacher. *Partner and peer support* is a further core asset.

Without such commitment, issues can arise around service replacement and workload, the drain on one's energy of the occasional 'problem' learner becomes a lonely business and the 'spin-offs' from one GP's educational activity for the rest of the team are much diminished.

There is a clear *human resource implication* for GP teaching, and the RCGP has been vocal in supporting the need to surpass the suggested increase in the number of GPs set out in *The NHS Plan*[13] because of their support for such roles. The constraints of the Medical Practices Committee and GP self-employed status have meant that most GP teachers have historically made *ad hoc* arrangements for their service replacement, but this cannot adequately release the GP or replace their role for patients if there is a substantive and recurrent teaching role. With the demise of restrictive ratios of GPs to patient population, emergence of PCTs and various personal medical services (PMS) schemes, the scope for salaried posts which include or compensate for an educational role appear much enhanced.

Financial resources have already been mentioned: these are essential both to pay for replacement GP time and for any infrastructure costs, including that of administrative time for liaison with patients and assistance with 'back of desk' learning, such as data collection for audit projects. Fees around the UK tend to vary with the type of learner, the number of students present, the extent to which the GP can teach while working, the level of supervision needed, the costs of providing physical kit such as computers or clinical equipment and additional payments for attendance by patients or by the GP. At the time of writing, there was no national agreement as to what the fees for teaching undergraduate medical students should be as the demands of different courses on GP teachers show considerable variation: the postgraduate training allowance is relatively consistent across deaneries, while other training roles depend on the nature of the commitment. One of the barriers to increasing the number of university-based GP tutors has been the mismatch between clinical and academic salaries, and another has been the disparity of 'fee-for-service' arrangements for payment of individual GPs. It may be that the merger of training monies for medicine, nursing and other NHS staff into common budgets held by workforce development confederations in England will alter this picture in the near future.[14]

Securing people and the money to pay them is one challenge, but the GP teacher also needs *appropriate skills*. Postgraduate GP training in the UK is greatly admired for the rigour of its requirements: in the 1996–2000 Teaching Quality Assurance exercise across higher education, the GP components of undergraduate medical courses were also frequently highly commended. This is due in part to the very explicit staff recruitment and development policies employed across general practice teachers of all types, and the direct links between a personal commitment to a teaching role and the responsibility for fulfilling that role. Secondary care colleagues involved with medical education often compare their own situations unfavourably, both recognising that their workforce of teachers is more anonymous and therefore less committed, and also that GP teachers have usually undertaken a systematic training for their teaching tasks.[15] This is particularly true for GP trainers, but is increasingly the case for undergraduate GP tutors as well, as more take up a substantive ongoing commitment to this role. Acquiring educational skills can of course be a basis for both professional accreditation and the gain of additional qualifications.

The need for staff development and support implies that another need of GP teachers is *professional support from more experienced colleagues*. The small critical mass of GPs involved with the RCGP at its inception might laugh ruefully at the idea of having anyone to help them develop their skills as educators, but there has been an exponential increase in both the amount of GP teaching activity and those resourcing it: in particular, core figures in deaneries and universities head up training cascades which induct new tutors and sustain others.

GP teachers also need *willing learners*. It is demotivating to prepare a practice for training and then not have a GP registrar for two years. Similarly, a weak or troublesome student, or a group of learners who have negative attitudes to general practice-based learning, can be very challenging. The culture of medical education and cooperation between secondary and primary care may be very important here in ensuring that students are not put off general practice before they have had any contact with the discipline, and early contact with primary care that is now appearing in many undergraduate programmes may also be important here.

Finally, and perhaps more than anything else, GP teachers *need to like helping people learn*. It is a truism to say that all GP educators are novices at the start.

Studies have shown that enthusiasm to educate, respect for the efforts of learners, good planning and preparation, and a willingness to evaluate are important start-up skills. The exact nature of the learner and the objectives determines what needs to be done in preparation, and the adage that 'a nice doctor is not necessarily a good doctor' applies to teaching: one can be well liked by students while teaching them poor technique. Nevertheless, it is also true that humiliating students will block their learning: challenge is valuable, but can only be truly effective if they also respect your views and are willing to hear what you are saying.

What are the benefits of being a GP teacher?

Some of these have been outlined already, but it is worth pointing out that many find their skills refreshed and improved: critical enquiry, evidence-based practice, communication skills and core factual knowledge may all be enhanced through one's involvement in teaching. These 'spin-offs' go broader than the specific content of the course taught as educational awareness alerts the practitioner to other areas of uncertainty. Learners will 'challenge' too, asking why and how one does certain things in practice. Beyond that, there are the benefits of the peer group sharing their expertise, the 'time out' of the front line and a considerable pride in seeing progress. The status of being a GP educator is recognised by many, and it is one of the few aspects of practice which most people consider to be valuable.

The role of the RCGP

Many of the GPs who teach and train, those who work as academics in higher education and those who act as continuing professional development (CPD) tutors are also Members or Fellows of the RCGP, and active in their faculties or local universities and vocational training (VT) schemes. The large number of quality awards from the RCGP involve active learning and educational leadership. Many of the core texts used in general practice education have come from College members; for example, Neighbour's *The Inner Apprentice*[16] or Fry *et al.*'s *Guide for Trainees*.[17]

As far back as the start of the College, foundation members were recognised as key contributors whose expert opinion on medical training was sought at a national level.[18] The MRCGP examination is associated with a string of educational publications. *A College Plan: priorities for the future*,[19] in providing an educational strategy for the 1990s, introduced for the first time higher professional education, called for more recognition and resources for research work and rationalisation of education in general practice, and set the scene for a much more broadly based educational role for the College.

The College has rewarded the contribution of those active in education and service through its Fellowships, and has chosen many educationalists as its leaders over its first half century. It therefore appears that there is a natural reciprocity between the RCGP and the role of GPs as teachers. Certainly educational activity is often associated with quality in practice, and quality is a consequence of educational engagement. We celebrate the development of the role of GPs as teachers: where would their patients, colleagues and the next generation of GPs be without them?

References

1 Jones R, Higgs R, de Angelis C *et al.* (2001) Changing face of medical curricula. *Lancet.* **357**: 699–703.

2 Wass V, Van der Vieuten C, Shatzer J *et al.* (2001) Assessment of clinical competence. *Lancet.* **357**: 945–9.

3 Howe A, Carter Y, Thomas K *et al.* (2000) *Undertaking Higher Research Degrees: some practical guidance.* Royal College of General Practitioners, London.

4 Carter Y and Jackson N (2002) *Guide to Education and Training for Primary Care.* Oxford University Press, Oxford.

5 Van Es JC, Melker RA de and Goosmann FCL (1983) *Characteristics of the General Practitioner: revised report on educational objectives of the Department of General Practice of the University of Utrecht.* Bohn, Scheltema and Holkema, Utrecht/Antwerpen. (In Dutch.)

6 Harris CM (1969) *General Practice Teaching of Undergraduates in British Medical Schools.* Reports from General Practice No. XI. Royal College of General Practitioners, London.

7 Byrne PS (1973) University departments of general practice and undergraduate teaching of general practice in the United Kingdom in 1972. *Journal of the Royal College of General Practitioners.* **23** (1): 1–12.

8 Howie JGR, Hannay DR and Stevenson JSK (1986) *The Mackenzie Report: general practice in the medical schools of the United Kingdom, 1986.* University of Edinburgh, Edinburgh.

9 Howe A (2000) Teaching in practice: a qualitative factor analysis of community-based teaching. *Medical Education.* **34** (9): 762–8.

10 Howe A and Hand C (2002) The challenge of doing things differently: one new medical school's vision of primary care education. *Education for Primary Care.* **13** (2): 205–321.

11 Gray RW, Carter YH, Hull SA *et al.* (2001) Characteristics of general practices involved in undergraduate medical training. *British Journal of General Practice.* **51**: 371–4.

12 Hesketh EA, Bagnall G, Buckley EG *et al.* (2001) A framework for developing excellence as a clinical educator. *Medical Education.* **35**: 555–64.

13 Department of Health (2000) *The NHS Plan: a plan for investment, a plan for reform.* The Stationery Office, London.

14 Percy D and Easmon C (2002) Education and training in the NHS in England. In: Carter Y and Jackson N (eds) *Guide to Education and Training for Primary Care.* Oxford University Press, Oxford.

15 Murray E, Jolly B and Modell M (1997) Can students learn clinical method in general practice? A randomised cross-over trial based on objective structured clinical examinations. *BMJ.* **315**: 920–3.

16 Neighbour R (1992) *The Inner Apprentice: an awareness-centred approach to vocational training for general practice.* Kluwer Academic Publishers, Dordrecht.

17 Fry J, Gambrill E, Godfrey M *et al.* (1989) *A Guide for Trainees in General Practice.* Heinemann, Oxford.

18 Rose FM and Cohen H (1948) *The Training of a Doctor: report of the BMA Medical Curriculum Committee.* Butterworth, London.

19 Royal College of General Practitioners (1990) *A College Plan: priorities for the future.* RCGP, London.

CHAPTER 10

The story of general practice postgraduate training and education

Steve Field

Ancient history of general practice education

The teaching of rational medicine has its origin in the Greek concepts of medicine, which combined scientific enquiry, applied theory and the belief in searching out knowledge for its own sake. In medieval Britain, Bede (731) described the church's central role in the development of medical knowledge and skills, but Latin medical and surgical texts such as the *Compendium Medicinae* (*c*.1240) and the *Rosa Anglica* (*c*.1314) were, however, only accessible to the few academic scholars, not to ordinary practitioners.[1]

The development of education, assessment and continuing education processes as we would now recognise them started with the medieval guilds. Apothecaries and barber-surgeons increased their strength and influence by forming themselves into guilds, while the foundation of the universities of Cambridge and Oxford in the fourteenth century generated a breed of 'elite' physicians who graduated with degrees and doctorates in medicine. The potent rivalry between apothecaries and physicians began then because the 'elite' and more academic physicians remained aloof while the apothecaries tended to be closer to the people. It was the apothecaries who stayed to care for the common inhabitants of London during the plague when physicians and their rich patients moved out to the country.

A hundred years after the formation of the College of Physicians, the apothecaries were granted a royal charter; the hostility between the groups continued. The term 'general practitioner' came into use in the early 1800s and the physicians continued their struggle to extend their dominance over the whole of the profession, but a turning point came in 1815 when the Society of Apothecaries was established by an Act of Parliament and led to a legal judgment that legally qualified GPs required the licentiateship of the Society of Apothecaries. A five-year apprenticeship was required and from 1834 all apprentices were required to pass an examination at the end of their training and submit a formal testimonial.

The first half of the nineteenth century also saw an increase in activity in medical education with the first publication of the *Lancet* (1832) and establishment of the Royal Society of Medicine (1805) and the Provincial Medical and Surgical Association in Worcester in 1832 (which later became the British Medical Association). There was even an Association of General Practitioners founded in 1833 and an attempt in the 1840s to establish a Royal College of General Practitioners.[2]

The effects of the Medical Acts of 1815 improved the regulation of the medical profession by establishing the General Medical Council and a minimum standard of medical education, but once qualified the doctor could legally work anywhere across the UK without any further education or qualification. The Medical Act of 1858 led to a further increase in standards by requiring a pass in medicine, surgery and midwifery in the final medical examination.

By the end of the nineteenth century the role of the GP had developed to be very similar to that of the family doctor of today. Many GPs of the time also developed special interests, working in their local hospitals as physicians or surgeons, but there was no additional training for the role. Early in the twentieth century, the National Health Insurance Act of 1911 brought with it a capitation-based service and the concept of patients being on the doctor's 'list'. Education and training did not, however, show any sign of development despite the publication of influential general practice books by authors including Sykes (*A Manual for General Practice*, 1927) and Le Fleming (*An Introduction to General Practice*, 1936).

The National Health Service was formed in 1948, a year that saw the publication of a BMA report, *The Training of a Doctor*, which is a landmark in general practice education because it identified the need for better education for GPs and the need for them to keep up to date (but by being taught by hospital specialists!). A later report in 1950 of a working party chaired by Lord Cohen proposed specific postgraduate training for GPs; neither report was adopted by the BMA as policy. No further progress was made until after considerable effort and political manoeuvring, the College of General Practitioners was founded on 19 November 1952.

Modern history

Foundation of the College of General Practitioners

The foundation of the College of General Practitioners in 1952 was the most significant event in the history of GP education in the UK. The College became the national focus for change and development, a position that it retains today in its 51st year.

On 21 January 1953, eight weeks after the Foundation Council of the College met for the first time, a Postgraduate Education and Regional Organisational Committee was formed. It quickly defined the difference between postgraduate education (the period between medical school and becoming a GP principal) and continuing medical education for the period after gaining a principal post in general practice. There was a trainee year available under the NHS, but there was no formal hospital training or the half-day release courses of the sort that we are familiar with today.[2] In the early 1950s, an experiment in GP training began in Inverness, while the Nuffield Provincial Hospitals Trust funded an early scheme in Wessex. The 1959 annual report of the College also included a brief description of a proposed 'postgraduate training for general practice in two years analogous to registrarships for the specialities'.

In 1961, the Platt Committee report led to junior hospital posts being regarded as training posts. In the same year, the College of General Practitioners published *Training for General Practice: a guide to non-clinical aspects*. Trainers received this paper positively but they were frustrated because the paper failed to address the needs of trainers who wished to develop the clinical aspects of their training. In 1965, the College published an influential policy on vocational training for general practice.[3] The case was made for formal training for all doctors before entry into general practice. It suggested a broad programme of training, including several hospital posts and time spent in a training practice. It was followed by a further report, *The Implementation of Vocational Training*.[4]

In 1968, the Royal Commission on Medical Education (known as the Todd Commission) recommended a change in the organisation of medical training to encompass a period of 'general professional training' followed by a period of specialist training. It also led to the establishment of Regional Advisors in General Practice. The College had pushed for training to be a minimum of four years' duration, including two years in supervised practice; while we continue to wait for the two-year GP training period to be implemented, the concept that general practice should be treated like the other specialities was accepted. The evidence from the RCGP was published as the *Report from General Practice No. 5*.[5] The strong educational leadership demonstrated by the College reinforced its role as the key force in developing postgraduate GP education across the UK. The next success, the appointment of the first two Regional Advisors in General Practice, George Swift in Wessex and Douglas Price in London, followed after considerable lobbying and by the Conference of Local Medical Committees accepting, in 1971, that vocational training 'should normally be mandatory for those wishing to be principals in general practice'. In order to take forward the consensus, in 1976, the College's Vocational Training Committee opened up to new members from the General Medical Services Committee (GMSC) of the British Medical Association. It was agreed that the new 'Joint Committee' would have an Honorary Joint Secretary provided by each of the parent bodies and a Chair that would alternate between them. The first Chairman was from the College: John Lawson. In addition to the founder members, representation is now drawn from other bodies including the Committee of General Practice Education Directors (COGPED), the Association of Course Organisers and from GP registrars.

Formation of the Joint Committee on Postgraduate Training for General Practice (JCPTGP)

The JCPTGP has had a massive effect on the development of postgraduate GP education since it was formed in 1976. The founding objective was to monitor the quality of general practice training. When the Vocational Training Regulations were introduced (as part of the NHS Acts), it was designated as the body responsible for assessing the training and experience of doctors applying for certificates of eligibility to practise as principals in the NHS. In 1994, the JCPTGP was confirmed as the Competent Authority under the European Directive 93/16/EEC. The 1997 NHS (Vocational Training for General Medical Practice) Regulations (and their 1998 equivalent regulations in Scotland and Northern Ireland) gave the JCPTGP the responsibility for approving all training posts for GP training both in hospitals and in training practices across the UK. The JCPTGP quality controls the deaneries' processes by a programme of accreditation visits to each deanery. By using its powers in a constructive and supportive way, the JCPTGP has brought about change that has resulted in an improvement in the quality of GP training across the whole of the UK.

Vocational training schemes become a reality

The first formal vocational training scheme was founded by College pioneers in Inverness in 1951. Schemes in Wessex and the West Midlands followed in the 1960s. Their success paved the way for schemes to be introduced across the UK, but it was not until 1976 that the UK Parliament approved legislation that required completion of vocational training for general practice before a doctor could become a GP principal. It was implemented in 1982. Doctors training to become GPs may train full time or on a part-time basis. They also have a choice between joining a VT scheme and constructing their own programme. The proportion of doctors on VT schemes is increasing because there are advantages over DIY programmes.

The length and content of the VT programmes are governed by the VT regulations which allow for programmes to include up to 24 months as a GP registrar and a minimum of 12 months in a hospital post. In the armed forces 18 months in general practice has been the normal practice for many years, but, in civilian practice, only a few doctors each year are able to spend 18 months in general practice. It was not possible at all until 2000 except for those doctors receiving extended training because they had failed an element of summative assessment. However, in April 2000 it was agreed that the budget for GP vocational training would move from the General Medical Services (GMS) budget to the Medical and Dental Education Levy (MADEL). This opened up opportunities for trainees to spend a larger part of their training in the primary care setting pursuing a particular learning need. Innovative placements in general practice now include academic links to universities and focused learning in subjects which include sexual health, child health, drug addiction and care of the homeless. The new arrangements were also designed to allow the directors of postgraduate general practice education to provide more opportunities for refresher training for doctors returning to general practice and for those who have trained abroad.

The introduction of assessment

Assessment of competence to practise as a GP was slow to receive support in the UK despite being introduced in Australia, Canada and America.[6]

For many years, the GP educational establishment focused on educational methods and developing educational programmes; the introduction of VT schemes was a triumph envied by the wider profession, but there was no compulsory end-point assessment of training. As a consequence, most trainees were awarded their JCPTGP certificate of satisfactory completion of vocational training with no assessment of their competence. Over the years 1989–92 the number of trainees who were refused a certificate at the end of their training was only 0.26%.[7]

The membership examination of the RCGP, introduced in 1965, was not compulsory (this continues to be the situation). The RCGP[8] proposed that the MRCGP examination should become the end-point assessment because the majority of trainees took the MRCGP exam at the end of their training. The fail rate was, however, over 25% and therefore doctors continued to become GP principals without sitting the MRCGP exam or having failed it.[9]

Despite these facts, there was little discussion in the profession about 'competence' to practise as a GP until the late 1980s, driven by Donald Irvine and Denis Pereira Gray who were active as Regional Advisors and had leadership roles in the RCGP. The suggestion was made that satisfactory completion of training only meant time served. Therefore after taking legal advice, the Chairs of the RCGP, the GMSC and JCPTGP stated in 1990 that the certificate of satisfactory completion of vocational training was a certificate of competence as opposed to a certificate of attendance.[10] Concerns also began to be raised that the public and the profession needed to be reassured about the standard of entry into general practice.[11] The JCPTGP eventually decided that all GP trainees should pass an objective test at the end of training after September 1996. It stated summative assessment would involve six elements: a test of factual knowledge; tests of problem solving; a submission of practical work; an evaluation of clinical skills; an evaluation of consulting skills and the trainer's overall assessment.[12]

The profession then entered a period of discussion and argument. The RCGP had held the view for many years that the MRCGP qualification should be held by all who become principals in general practice. There was also support from a significant proportion of the education and medico-political establishment. This was demonstrated in an editorial in *Postgraduate Education for General Practice* in 1993 by Bahrami,[13] which stated that 'the present MRCGP examination (with some modifications) would be ideal'. There was, however, sufficient resistance from some quarters to make its use impossible.[14]

It was therefore decided that a national system of summative assessment be introduced which would not be the MRCGP examination in its entirety. The JCPTGP determined that there would be four components of the new summative assessment system, known then as the 'UK Regional Advisors Package'. They were a multiple-choice questionnaire, a written submission of practical work, an assessment of consulting skills and the final component was to be the structured trainers report.[15] An exemption was also made for doctors who gained a satisfactory pass in the MRCGP examination's MCQ paper. It was determined that in order to obtain a satisfactory completion of the GP training certificate, GP registrars would have to pass all four modules.

Summative assessment was therefore introduced by the Conference of Regional Advisors across the UK as a professionally led assessment system in 1996. Its gestation and its ultimate introduction were surrounded by controversy, but in 1998 the UK Government finally introduced the VT regulations which made it a legal requirement for all trainees.[16–18]

Summative assessment has had both positive and negative effects. Campbell and Murray[19] demonstrated that prior to its introduction, trainers did occasionally fail to recognise incompetent trainees. Audit and clinical effectiveness have also become an established part of the curriculum and the use of video in the teaching and assessment of consulting skills has also increased.[20] There has, however, been criticism that summative assessment took trainees away from other educational activities and increased the pressure on them during their 'short' training year.[21,22] There was also debate about the validity of the approved system and the unnecessary duplication of assessments that resulted in GP registrars having to prepare for both summative assessment and the MRCGP examination. The GP registrars also felt that the description of being 'minimally competent' was derisory.[18] The vast majority of GP registrars will pass summative assessment without having to apply for additional support and training. By January 2002, 6384 doctors had satisfactorily completed summative assessment since its introduction in 1996. The average failure rate was only 3.78% and most trainees passed after an additional period of training.

Ever since summative assessment was introduced, GP registrars, trainers, course organisers and directors of postgraduate general practice education have complained about the 'waste of time' spent during the GP training year preparing for two different systems of assessing videotapes of consultations: one for summative assessment, the other for the MRCGP examination. The RCGP eventually succeeded in gaining approval for its video assessment of consulting skills[23] and, since summer 2001, a single route through both summative assessment and the MRCGP examination has been available. GP registrars were permitted to prepare a single tape that once submitted to their deanery office is passed through the MRCGP assessment process. A pass (or pass with merit) is accepted as a pass for summative assessment purposes. The single-route option has proved to cut down the time that a GP registrar has to spend on preparing their videotape, which frees up time to devote to their other learning needs.

Approved alternative methods of assessing the required competencies have also been put forward. The trainees have continued to claim that they are confused by the proliferation of assessment instruments, their requirements and the different timetables used in the deaneries across the UK.[24]

Changes in funding: the 'MADEL transfer'

Training to be a GP has always been a compromise between education, training and providing a service to patients. GP training has also appeared to be of secondary importance in the UK to the training of specialists. There was also a feeling across the profession that GP training was stuck in a time warp.[25] There were many suggestions on how it could be improved but the regulations were not changed.[26,27]

In 1995, ambitious recommendations were proposed by the then Chief Medical Officer, Sir Kenneth Calman, in the supplement to the main report of his working group on specialist medical training, *Hospital Doctors: training for the future*.[28] The supplement considered the implications for general medical practice of the 'Calmanisation' of specialist hospital training. Calman recommended that recognised resources should be transferred from the General Medical Services budget to the postgraduate deans' budget. There was no change.

A new 'GP Registrar Scheme' was launched in March 2000.[29] The launch heralded a fundamental change in the funding arrangements for VT that aimed to deliver a more flexible approach to training within the standards set by the JCPTGP across the UK. The changes resulted from a shift of the budget for GP vocational training from the GMS budget to the MADEL. The implementation of the new arrangements was made possible by unprecedented collaboration between the Department of Health, the RCGP, COGPED and the General Practitioners Committee of the BMA. The change became known as the 'MADEL Transfer'. This flexibility has led to the development of a number of innovative service and academic training schemes. Early indications are that the schemes have been successful with the first GP registrars passing their membership examinations and obtaining higher awards. Academic papers are beginning to be published by the trainees and some are considering academic careers.

The MADEL Transfer also brought about a radical change in the way GP trainees were recruited. Selection for GP training became the responsibility of the Directors of Postgraduate General Practitioner Education (DsPGPE) rather than individual trainers. The basis of the new system was a nationally agreed list of core competencies, against which candidates' performance was assessed. The new processes were also consistent with the principles of equal opportunities.

Postgraduate Medical Education and Training Board (PMETB)

In July 2000, the Department of Health published *The NHS Plan*.[30] It announced that the JCPTGP and the Specialist Training Authority were to be abolished and replaced by a new regulatory body provisionally called the Medical Education Standards Board (later renamed the Postgraduate Medical Education and Training Board). The Department of Health subsequently published its consultation paper *Postgraduate Medical Education and Training: the Medical Education Standards Board*.[31] The objective of the new body was described as 'to ensure that patients' interests and the service needs of the NHS are aligned with the development of the curriculum and the approval of training programmes for medical specialists and general practitioners'. It was proposed that the new Board would supervise all postgraduate medical education, including general practice. It would set curricula and approve training programmes working through the postgraduate deaneries. It would also issue certificates showing that individual doctors had reached the required standard at the end of training.

The arrangements for regulating postgraduate medical education had developed in a piecemeal way since Victorian times and there were large variations between the regulatory systems for training specialists and GPs. The Department of Health had also grown wary of the role that the Royal Colleges played in the delivery of postgraduate medical training. High-profile cases where a Royal College had removed education approval from hospital posts without considering the adverse effect on patient care were seen as the catalyst for the Department of Health's action. Concerns were also raised about the wider accountability of the Royal Colleges and their decision-making processes.

The consultation document provoked a heated debate across the profession. The proposals were seen by many as a direct threat to the autonomy of the Royal Colleges. The BMA called for a rethink and Denis Pereira Gray, Chairman of the Academy of Royal Colleges, considered, (in a *British Medical Journal* [BMJ] editorial) 'the medical profession to be under unprecedented attack' and predicted that changes would 'transform medicine into a controlled profession'.[32]

The heat of battle drew attention away from the real need to modernise what had become a fragmented and poorly designed system. Change was needed and there were some very sound ideas suggested in the Department of Health's consultation document. It also offered the opportunity for general practice training to be considered in equal standing to specialist training.

The proposal to rationalise the quality assurance mechanisms for training placements was well received by the deaneries but was perceived as a major threat to the Royal Colleges. The prevailing situation where inspection visits to trusts by many different bodies at different times, to different training grades and different specialities is absurd. Change is needed; the new PMETB should be able to deliver it. The RCGP, working through its Hospital Recognition Committee (HRC) and the JCPTGP, has had a massive impact at senior house officer (SHO) level that has ensured that the SHO placements have GP-orientated education and access to half-day release courses. The HRC has also been proactive in approving and disapproving appropriate SHO posts for trainee GPs and has worked collaboratively with the Hospital Recognition Committees of the specialist Colleges. In the future, GPs should be involved at all levels in the selection and approval of the posts for GP vocational training. The JCPTGP system of visiting deaneries to ensure that they are adequately quality assuring their placements and GP programmes seems to be a sensible way forward. The establishment of the PMETB should empower the RCGP to become the standard setter for GP vocational training, becoming responsible for both the curriculum design and assessment of trainees alongside its sister specialist Royal Colleges. It is an opportunity to unite the profession and absorb what is good in summative assessment into a new, unified assessment system. A unified system could also enable the timing of assessments to be more appropriate and facilitate education and the passage of the trainee through the training programme.

In the latter part of 2000, the Chief Medical Officer in England announced a review of the SHO grade. An initial period of intense consultation (running concurrently with the PMETB consultation) was followed by many months of eager expectation. The review will radically alter training for general practice by recommending that all doctors go through a foundation period of two years, comprising the existing pre-registration house officer year and a year of basic professional training time in a variety of placements at SHO level followed by a period of basic specialist training in one of eight specialities or general practice.

There will also be opportunities for specialists to spend time learning and experiencing primary care during the foundation period.

If the Department of Health delivers the changes proposed in the PMETB consultation and in the review of the SHO grade, then there should be an opportunity to radically change and modernise the structure of GP training in the UK to meet the challenges of the 'new NHS'.

The General Medical Council publishes *Good Medical Practice* guidance

In 1995, the GMC launched its significant guidance document *Good Medical Practice.*[33] It defined the basic principles of good medical practice and as a consequence has had a major impact on the development of medical practice, education and continuing professional development in the UK. To date, the guidance has been updated on three occasions. It has become a central factor in curriculum development, assessment and revalidation by describing what is expected of a GP. The GMC has also had a major effect on the modernisation of the undergraduate medical curriculum and the pre-registration house officer (PRHO) year. Since the publication of *The New Doctor* in 1997,[34] PRHOs have been able to be placed in general practice, but, because of the perception of underfunding of training practices, opportunities have been few.

A gaze into the future

The NHS Plan,[30] published in 2000, represents the Government's ten-year programme of investment and reform. The vision is for prompt, convenient, high-quality healthcare services which treat patients as partners. It aims to produce improved health outcomes, particularly for the poorest in society. This modernisation programme puts primary care in the pivotal role. The Government also claims that NHS staff are their greatest asset and are the key to the reform process. It has made a commitment to put a greater share of new NHS funding into the training of healthcare professionals. While there are plans to produce a net increase of 15 000 GPs and consultants by 2008,[35] the significant shortage of GPs and other staff currently working in primary care puts their modernisation plans at risk. More health professionals equipped with appropriate knowledge and skills are needed. To support this, a radical review of GP training as part of a larger review of the training of health professionals who work in primary care is urgently needed.

In 2001, WONCA Europe* started a wide consultation process to produce a consensus statement to define the discipline of general practice, the professional tasks and the core competencies required of GPs. The final definition was published and formally endorsed by the RCGP in June 2002.[36] The definition reinforced the view that general practice is an academic and scientific discipline with its own educational content, research, evidence base and clinical activity, and a clinical speciality orientated to primary care.

The definition defined six core competencies essential to the discipline:[36]

1 primary care management
2 person-centred care
3 specific problem-solving skills
4 comprehensive approach
5 community orientation
6 holistic modelling.

It went on to say that the competent practitioner would implement these competencies in three areas: clinical tasks, communicating with patients and management of the practice. It also suggested that there were three background fundamental features:

- contextual – using the context of the person, the family, the community and their culture
- attitudinal – based on the doctor's professional capabilities, values and ethics
- scientific – adopting a critical and research-based approach to practice and maintaining this through learning and quality improvement.

Despite the different healthcare systems across Europe, these newly defined competencies chime well with British general practice and the 'new NHS'. The work will help to inform a review of GP education and training that should lead to a radical change in the arrangements for VT that began in 2002, when the JCPTGP published a paper on the future of GP vocational training. It was written by the RCGP's Vocational Training Working Group following a wide consultation involving stakeholders.[37] It put forward a framework of principles and an 'outcomes-based' approach in which objectives were clearly defined (*see* Box 10.1).

The JCPTGP paper also determined that the education should be based in the community and learner-centred to mirror the patient-centred approach in clinical practice. Work has begun on drawing up recommendations for changes in the regulatory framework for GP vocational training to implement the above principles. The RCGP has also started work on the design of a new curriculum

---

*WONCA Europe – The European Society of General Practice/Family Medicine (the regional organisation of the World Organisation of Family Doctors).

Box 10.1 Principles for the future of GP Vocational Education[37]

- The educational programme should be based on the key features of learner-centred, adult professional education and so be flexible in terms of content and length.
- The educational programme should focus on the provision, by appropriately trained GPs working with other healthcare disciplines in a general practice setting, of the best quality care for patients in the NHS.
- The programme should be based in general practice, supervised throughout by an educational facilitator (GP trainer) with carefully planned attachments in secondary and community care.
- The importance of the relationship between the learner and education facilitator is accepted but the paper recognises the need to explore and consider other models to address, among other issues, the problem of educational capacity.
- Regular relevant assessment is important not only to confirm educational progress but to assure patients of the competence of doctors at the point of certification (entitlement to enter independent practice).

---

and structure for GP vocational education based on the principles defined by its Vocational Training Working Group, the WONCA definition of general practice and the GMC's Good Medical Practice guidance.

And finally

The story of postgraduate education and training for general practice is entwined in the story of the development of the general practitioner from ancient times to the present day. It is, however, in the last 50 years that the most dramatic developments in the structure and regulation of training programmes for general practice have occurred. This has been to a great extent due to strong professional leadership. The next 50 years will also require strong leadership to ensure that opportunities are taken to produce the best quality education and training for doctors wishing to become GPs and as a result improve the quality of care provided for all patients.

Acknowledgements

I would like to acknowledge the extraordinary efforts that Professor Denis Pereira Gray has made to document the history of the RCGP. His book *Forty Years On: the story of the first forty years of the Royal College of General Practitioners,* published in 1992, has not only been a valuable source for this chapter but it has stimulated me to seek out and read more about the history of general practice and the College. Finally, thank you to Lynn who has once more been generous in her time and tolerance in reading and re-reading the manuscript.

References

1 Cule J (1980) *A Doctor for the People*. Update, London.

2 Pereira Gray D (1992) *Forty Years On: the story of the first forty years of the Royal College of General Practitioners*. Royal College of General Practitioners, London.

3 College of General Practitioners (1965) *Reports from General Practice No. 1*. CGP, London.

4 Royal College of General Practitioners (1967) *The Implementation of Vocational Training*. RCGP, London.

5 College of General Practitioners (1966) *Report from General Practice No. 5*. CGP, London.

6 Wakeford R (1990) *International Background in the Examination for Membership of the Royal College of General Practitioners (MRCGP)*. Occasional paper 46. Royal College of General Practitioners, London.

7 Campbell LM (1997) The development of summative assessment for vocational trainees in general practice [MD thesis]. University of Glasgow, Glasgow.

8 Royal College of General Practitioners (1988) *Policy on MRCGP*. RCGP, London.

9 Royal College of General Practitioners (1985) *Quality in General Practice*. Policy statement 2. RCGP, London.

10 Irvine D, Gray DJP and Bogle IG (1990) Vocational training: the meaning of 'satisfactory completion' [letter]. *British Journal of General Practice*. **40**: 434.

11 Joint Committee on Postgraduate Training for General Practice (1991) *Vocational Training for General Practice*. JCPTGP, London.

12 JCPTGP (1993) *Report of the Summative Assessment Working Party*. Joint Committee on Postgraduate Training for General Practice, London.

13 Bahrami J (1993) Assessment of vocational training: the present and future. *Postgraduate Education for General Practice*. **4** (3): 168–73.

14 Haslam D (1998) Why did the examination need to change? In: Moore R (ed.) *The MRCGP Examination: a guide for candidates and teachers*. Royal College of General Practitioners, London.

15 Johnson N, Hasler J, Toby J *et al*. (1996) Content of a trainer's report for summative assessment in general practice: views of trainers. *British Journal of General Practice*. **46**: 135–9.

16 Benett I (1995) The concerns of trainers and course organisers about summative assessment in the North West Region. *Education for General Practice*. **6**: 322–5.

17 Hayden J (1996) Summative assessment: threat or opportunity? *British Journal of General Practice*. **46**: 132–3.

18 Field SJ (1998) The MRCGP examination and summative assessment. In: Moore R (ed.) *The MRCGP Examination: a guide for candidates and teachers.* Royal College of General Practitioners, London.

19 Campbell LM and Murray TS (1996) Summative assessment of vocational trainees: results of a three-year study. *British Journal of General Practice.* **46**: 411–14.

20 Field SJ and Skelton JR (1998) The first year of summative assessment in the West Midlands Deanery: a questionnaire survey of the views of trainers and course organisers. *Education for General Practice.* **9**: 422–9.

21 Downey P (1997) Letter. *Education for General Practice.* **8**: 264–5.

22 Tegner H (1997) Summative assessment: a front-line perspective. *Education for General Practice.* **8**: 95–100.

23 Tate P, Foulkes J, Neighbour R *et al.* (1999) Assessing physicians' interpersonal skills via videotaped encounters: a new approach for the Royal College of General Practitioners Membership Examination. *Journal of Health Communication.* **4**: 143–52.

24 Personal Communication, National Summative Assessment Board, London.

25 Bain J (1996) Vocational training: the end or the beginning? *British Journal of General Practice.* **46**: 328–33.

26 Hayden J, Styles WMcN, Grant J *et al.* (1996) Developing vocational training for general practice: a system for the future. *Education for General Practice.* **7**: 1–7.

27 Elwyn GJ, Smail SA and Edwards AGK (1998) Is general practice in need of a career structure? *BMJ.* **317**: 731–3.

28 Department of Health (Calman K, Chairman) (1995) *Hospital Doctors: training for the future.* The Report of the Working Group on Specialist Registrar Training. (Supplementary report by the working groups commissioned to consider the implications for general medical practice, overseas doctors and academic and research medicine arising from the principal report, pp. 1–19.) DoH, London.

29 Department of Health (2000) *The GP Registrar Scheme: vocational training for general medical practice – the UK guide.* DoH, London.

30 Department of Health (2000) *The NHS Plan.* DoH, London.

31 Department of Health (2000) *Postgraduate Medical Education and Training: the Medical Education Standards Board.* DoH, London.

32 Pereira Gray D (2002) Deprofessionalising doctors? *BMJ.* **324**: 627–8.

33 General Medical Council (1995) *Good Medical Practice.* GMC, London.

34 GMC (1997) The New Doctor. Recommendations of General Clinical Training. GMC, London. www.gmc-uk.org/med_ed/newdoc.htm

35 Department of Health (2002) *Delivering the NHS Plan.* DoH, London.

36 WONCA Europe (2002) *The European Definition of General Practice/Family Medicine.* The European Society of General Practice/Family Medicine (WONCA Europe), Barcelona.

37 Joint Committee on Postgraduate Training for General Practice (2002) *The Future of GP Vocational Training.* JCPTGP, London.

CHAPTER 11

The creation and achievements of the RCGP

Denis Pereira Gray

Anniversaries are times for celebration, for looking back and learning lessons for the future. Fiftieth anniversaries are so special that they are called golden jubilees. Colleges, like marriages, need to celebrate half a century, a tangible measure of success.

It is hard now, in 2003, to think ourselves back over 50 years ago, although it is still well within the lifetime of a single doctor. So much has changed, so many systems are different, that it is quite easy to take for granted policies and practices that had to be fought for and were sometimes hard won.

The state of general practice in 1952

The word 'crisis' is overused, but it is appropriate for the state of general practice in 1952 in Britain. The facts speak for themselves and added up to a disaster scenario. Indeed, general practice did collapse at about this time in the USA and had to be reinvented as 'family medicine' in 1969.

The absence of training

In 1952, there was no training available for general practice. Indeed, the very idea that training was needed was the view of a small minority, although it had, to the great credit of the BMA, been proposed in the then recent Cohen reports.[1,2]

In 1952, there was not even a pre-registration year, although that, too, had been proposed by the Goodenough Committee.[3] This meant that medical students, on qualifying, could go straight into general practice without any hospital experience as a doctor and without any training for general practice.

Excluded from the universities

General practice had been excluded from the universities. There were no university-based research programmes led by primary care staff and there was not, until 1963, a professor of general practice anywhere in the world. University careers for general practitioners did not exist.

Apart from the dearth of postgraduate education, the undergraduate medical course lacked any significant general practice teaching, even though about half of all medical students would go on to be GPs. In 1953, only three medical schools ensured that all their students received any general practice teaching at all and two of these provided a single day![4]

Professional isolation

GPs were professionally isolated. The NHS contract of 1948 paid NHS GPs at that time wholly through a capitation fee, i.e. simply by the number of patients registered, at a flat rate per patient.

The good effect of this was that it helped to make that generation of doctors very patient-centred. The bad side of that contract was that it made GPs intensely competitive and they rarely shared ideas between themselves, let alone taught each other good practice. The other serious adverse effect of that contract was it guaranteed underinvestment, as there was a powerful perverse incentive not to invest in the practice.

Status

GPs had low status inside and outside the medical profession, most sharply expressed by the late Lord Moran, who was Dean of St Mary's Hospital Medical School and President, for many years, of the Royal College of Physicians of London. In giving evidence to the Royal Commission on Doctors' and Dentists' Remuneration, he was asked if consultants and GPs were equal. He said in 1956:[5]

> I say emphatically 'No'! Could anything be more absurd? I was Dean of St Mary's Medical School for 25 years ... all the people of outstanding merit, with few exceptions, aimed to get on the staff. There was no other aim and it was a ladder off which some of them fell. How can you say that the people who get to the top of the ladder are the same people who fall off it? It seems to me so ludicrous.

Lord Moran's ladder became notorious for the founding generation of the RCGP and has remained as a challenge. There was, however, some truth in Lord Moran's aphorism. Young doctors who wanted intellectual challenge and who wanted to be formally trained in medicine were drawn to specialist medicine, which alone offered high-quality extended medical training over years.

The founders of the College

The Section of General Practice of the Royal Society of Medicine was established in 1950.[6] Its significance was greater than the number of doctors involved. I believe it was a dress rehearsal for the College and it gave confidence to those involved.

The Section elected George Abercrombie, who had previously served as a Captain in the Royal Navy, as President with William Pickles as a Vice President. It was therefore no surprise when Abercrombie emerged two years later as the first Chairman of Council of the new College and after that William Pickles became the first President.

John Hunt and Fraser Rose emerged as the two key GP leaders. They were the two leading founders. Fraser Rose, an NHS GP from Preston, was the more senior medical politician, well established in the BMA. His classic memorandum of 1951, arguing for a College, was printed in full in *Forty Years On: the story of the first forty years of the Royal College of General Practitioners.*[7] John Hunt, a London GP in private practice, first met Rose in October 1951.

The two joined together to work for the founding of a College of General Practitioners. They were complementary and neither could have succeeded alone. Hunt had the personality and all the drive and contacts, but a College which would principally consist of NHS GPs needed an NHS GP leader and someone who could secure BMA support, or at least avoid BMA opposition. Their joint letter, with Rose as the first author, was published in October 1951 in the *Lancet* and *BMJ.*[8] Two weeks later two memoranda, one by Rose[9] and the other by Hunt,[10] were also published in the *BMJ.*

This led to the formation of a multidisciplinary Steering Committee which was the key group which made it all happen. It prepared the ground for a College of General Practitioners. The group first met in February 1952. It consisted of five GPs and five consultants. Sir Henry Willink, a former Minister of Health, was Chairman.

It was an extremely effective group. It took careful soundings and identified the powerful players in medicine, notably the then three existing English-based medical Royal Colleges, which were firmly hostile to a general practitioner College.

Sir Russell Brain's letter,[11] written on behalf of those three Colleges, was republished in *Forty Years On.* He wrote, on 11 January 1952, that these three specialist Royal Colleges had decided that they: 'Would not be able to support in any way an organisation which aimed at establishing another College ... I can say this with confidence because this very point has just been settled by the three Royal Colleges jointly in connection with another matter!'

Given that similar objections had thwarted proposals to found a College of General Practitioners in the 1840s,[12] careful plans and outstanding leadership were needed. General practice produced it.[13] After taking skilled legal advice, the proposed new College was established by the Steering Committee in *secret* on 19 November 1952.[14] The Steering Committee Report was then released in December 1952.[15] Thus the formation of the new College presented the world with a *fait accompli*.

Critically, the new College's appeal to ordinary NHS GPs in the UK to join, and pay to join, was successful. Two thousand joined in six months.[14] The College was launched and was secure by the summer of 1953, when branches, called faculties, were forming all round the British Isles and, soon, overseas as well.

Lessons to be learned

Crises can generate their own solutions

The first conclusion is that the College was formed as a direct result of the crisis in the medical profession and the weak and unsatisfactory position of general practice, especially the imbalance between generalist and specialist practice which had developed.

One trigger was the Collings Report,[16] which described a pattern of practice which was unacceptable. The solutions were either to abolish it or to reform it. The College was an organisational solution to the crisis in morale. The College was formed by those who believed in general practice and who were determined to reform it.

Linking enthusiasts

The second conclusion about the foundation of the College was that it brought together for the first time a group of enthusiastic GPs who did believe passionately in their job and who were prepared to work extremely hard to develop it. They worked together to develop, first systems of education and then research. The College has continued to function as a focal point for enthusiasts ever since and has, as the General Practice Steering Committee[15] correctly foresaw, become the repository of information about the craft.

Leadership

In 1952, every leadership post in British medicine was held by a hospital specialist and it was simply assumed that this was the natural order of things.

It was certainly not a subject for discussion or debate because specialist superiority was widely accepted and formed a fundamental part of the medical profession at that time. Indeed, this can be seen as an extension of the hierarchical structure of the medical profession, first established by the Medical Act 1858 and symbolised neatly by the hierarchy: LRCP (general practitioner), MRCP (qualified specialist) and FRCP (specialist leader). Quite apart from the culture, there were no GP leaders available.

The Second World War enabled a group of GP leaders to emerge, and in the various armed forces through the crisis of a World War. For the first time a group of GPs learnt strategic thinking, particularly those who reached the rank of Lieutenant-Colonel or above, to command and to achieve change under difficult circumstances. The new College used this new expertise with a Naval Captain as Chairman of Council, an army brigadier as the first Honorary Treasurer and several Lieutenant-Colonels in leadership roles, such as the first Honorary Editor. Such men, and it was a predominantly masculine group, accepted authority, could handle authority and could take decisions swiftly.

The College strategy

The College made swift progress by four main means:

- surveys and publications
- advocacy, through the organisation
- setting professional standards
- empowerment of individual GPs.

Surveys and publications

The College's early strategy was to survey and publish. For example, its survey on undergraduate medical education was published in the *BMJ*.[4] It stimulated reform by exposing the position through publications.

Advocacy for general practice

A major strategy for the College was advocacy, through the College as an organisation. Authorities were not necessarily unsympathetic and many of the chief medical officers in the Department of Health, from William Jamieson onwards and especially Sir George Godber, were sympathetic.

Setting standards

The third strand of the College's policy was to define standards in the field. Clinical practice in general practice was ripe for this and it was a field in which the medical Royal Colleges, and therefore the new College, had legitimacy.

An examination for entry to the College itself was highly controversial, but was successfully introduced as early as 1965. Later through Fellowship by Assessment introduced in 1989,[17] and Membership by Assessment introduced in 1999,[18] the College took control of standard setting for individual GPs on the basis of measuring performance.

Through the Quality in Practice Award,[19] the College reached out beyond the individual practitioner and set standards for primary healthcare teams.

Empowerment of GPs

Finally, the College consistently used its authority to value, welcome, reward, encourage and thus empower GPs when they did things well. A whole series of awards and prizes were introduced. As a result, the achievements of the discipline became better recognised through the successes of some of its leading practitioners.

Less publicly, but even more important, was the personal individual encouragement given by the early leaders to any GP who sought help or advice or who was ready to participate in the new enterprise.

The College's main achievements

The College's main achievements in its first 50 years can be summarised in a single theme. It has contributed, and done more than any other single organisation, to develop an academic discipline of general practice. It has done this through 12 key steps (*see* Box 11.1). These have been determined on evidence, outside the College, of effectiveness.

(1) 1954 – College research units

As the College was formed before any of the departments of general practice, it was the early generator of, and advocate for, general practice research. Early College-based GP researchers developed the key tools of clinical research in primary care: the age–sex register[20] and the disease register.[21]

The College research units were remarkably successful. The Birmingham Unit, led by Donald Crombie and Robin Pinsent, soon led the national morbidity

Box 11.1 The College's 12 key steps to developing an academic discipline of general practice

1	College research units: Birmingham, Manchester, Peaslake, Leigh	1954
2	Publishing and editing the world's first scientific journal in general practice, founding it in 1958 and gaining acceptance in *Index Medicus* in 1961 – the first primary care journal in the world to be so recognised. (*Journal of the [Royal] College of General Practitioners*, now *the British Journal of General Practice*)	1958–61
3	Establishing GPs in universities and supplying, through a Council member, the world's first Chair of General Practice and later as many as 12 other professors	1963–2002
4	Developing vocational training for general practice	1965–77
5	Establishing the first examination in general practice in Europe: the MRCGP	1965
6	Establishing GPs as authors: GP books, written as individuals and through the College. Publishing academic manuscripts: the *Occasional Papers*	1972–76
7	Establishing the first Patient Group within any medical Royal College	1985
8	Establishing the first high-quality performance measurement of general practice, in the setting of general practice: Fellowship by Assessment	1989
9	Establishing research general practices, now NHS funded	1994
10	Establishing Membership by Assessment of Performance	1999
11	Establishing the first international examination: the MRCGP International	2000
12	Establishing an assessment for primary healthcare teams: the Quality in Practice Award	2000

surveys in general practice, and the Manchester Research Unit, led by Clifford Kay, undertook the largest survey in the world of women on the Pill.[22] Although the conduct of most primary care research has now rightly moved to the universities, the College remains a major advocate; for example, in its evidence to a Select Committee of Parliament.[23]

(2) 1961 – College journal: the first scientific journal of general practice in the world

The core of the discipline is the body of knowledge, and in science this means knowledge published in peer-reviewed journals and recognised internationally.

But in 1952, there was a major problem. There was no peer-reviewed journal for general practice anywhere in the world, and so any GP publishing an original article was forced to do so either in a specialist medical journal devoted to another field or in one of the few general medical journals like the *Lancet* or *BMJ*. As early as 1958, the new College identified this need and solved it by establishing its own peer-reviewed journal.

The early newsletter of the College, *Between Ourselves*, was developed into a scientific journal in 1958 by the founding editor, RMS McConaghey (Mac), a GP in Dartmouth, Devon. Within the remarkably short time of only three years, this journal was recognised by *Index Medicus* in the United States and so became the first primary care journal worldwide to be accepted scientifically.

Pereira Gray, in the 1988 McConaghey Memorial Lecture,[24] interpreted this event, coupled with other events such as the emergence of clinical books written by GPs in 1961, as marking the establishment of general practice as an academic discipline. It happened in Britain as the British College of General Practitioners, and especially its journal, was at that time literally leading the world.

(3) 1963 – Fostering the entry of GPs in universities: the first professor of general practice in the world

Early statements from the College expressed aspirations for GP lectureships, but soon the aim crystallised on Chairs. The first Chair of General Practice in the world came at the University of Edinburgh in 1963 and was filled by a member of the Council of the College. The relatively small Council of the College went on to supply the first Chair of General Practice in England, the first Chair in Canada, the first Chair in Ireland and the first postgraduate Chair of General Practice in Britain as well as several others. This is strong evidence of a leader group, encouraging and empowering its members to scale new heights.

(4) 1965 – Vocational training for general practice

Although as early as 1953 the College was surveying undergraduate education, a critical strategic decision was made as early as the 1950s to concentrate primarily on postgraduate training. A small number of far-sighted leaders grasped the essential fact that until there was formal, postgraduate-specific vocational training for general practice there would be very little hope of seriously raising clinical standards.

The work of the College in the 1960s can therefore be seen as almost a single-issue charity and many major speeches, eponymous lectures and College publications of this time mostly sought to set out the reasons for VT, the ways in which it could be organised and the fostering and reporting of numerous pilots. In 1965, the College published the first of its Reports from General Practice, *Special Vocational Training for General Practice*.[25] This little booklet, priced at five shillings (25p), was to prove extraordinarily influential.

Another publication in 1967, entitled *The Implementation of Vocational Training*,[26] neatly illustrated how quickly the College was moving on from advocacy to implementation.

In 1976, Parliament approved compulsory GP training in the 1977 NHS Act. This was implemented in stages, culminating in 1982, by which time every future GP was completing a pre-registration year in the hospital service and then three years of planned VT for general practice, i.e. four years full time after qualification.

The achievement of three years of VT, mandated by law as early as 1976, must rank as one of the main achievements of the College.

(5) 1965 – Developing an examination in general practice

Medical education and training serve a purpose, and that purpose is better standards of patient care.

Educational theory demands that assessment is an integral part of the educational process.[27] It was therefore logical to introduce a professional examination in general practice itself in order to mark successful completion of a programme of VT for general practice. This was done in 1965 for the first time in Europe and the MRCGP examination has attracted almost 2000 candidates in some years.[28]

(6) 1972 – General practitioner writings: books and *Occasional Papers*

There had been a few books written by GPs over the years, e.g. Pickles,[29] but it was not until after the College was founded that there was a real flow. In 1961 there were two clinical books written by GPs who were College activists on what were prime general practice topics.[30,31] Then in 1972 came the College's own book, *The Future General Practitioner: learning and teaching*,[32] an educational classic setting out a general practice curriculum for the first time. Two years later, Kay wrote *Oral Contraceptives and Health*[22] for the College.

In 1976, the Editorial Board of the College journal decided, after a considerable debate, to introduce the *Occasional Papers*, which were to be separate academic publications. By 1997, there had been 78 published and the series was paying its own way. No other College published such academic publications.

These developments helped to foster the spate of GP books which have now appeared. In the 1980s, the College started publishing books in its own right.

(7) 1985 – A Patient Group within the College

The RCGP was the first medical Royal College to establish a Patient Group within the College, with a lay Chair attending Council and later the Council Executive Committee. Even in 2003, 18 years later, this has not happened in other medical Royal Colleges.

(8) 1989 – Fellowship of the College by Assessment

In 1989, the College foresaw that education would move towards continuing professional development, which would become increasingly performance based. Sooner or later performance would need to be assessed in the setting where patients were seen.

The central task of the College is to foster 'the highest possible standards of general practice'. Defining those in measurable terms was achieved in 1989 when it was agreed to offer Fellowship, by a new route, to those who achieved it. The College was the first medical Royal College to achieve this.

Fellowship by Assessment was another world first for the College and showed that medical performance in the broadest of all the branches of medicine could be rigorously assessed though a system including annual review of the standards. There are now about 250 GPs who have passed this exceptionally high standard of clinical care.[33]

(9) 1994 – Research general practices

Research in general practice outside universities was crippled because the GP NHS contract was research free, unlike the considerable support the NHS gave research in hospitals. A new entity was needed through which funding could be routed.

The College invented the model in 1994, using subscription income. Within three years, one NHS regional authority alone had committed over a million pounds to NHS research and development practices. There are now NHS R&D practices all over the UK. The College's evidence to the House of Lords in 1995 on general practice research was published by the House of Lords through Her Majesty's Stationery Office (HMSO).

(10) 1999–2000 – Membership of the College by Assessment of Performance

As a direct result of the success of the College's Fellowship by Assessment came logically the extension to Membership by Assessment. The principles were the same, i.e. assessment in the setting of the practice against published previously agreed standards and assessed by peers and patients. This resolved two outstanding problems: the definition of a clinical standard for working members, and the complaining by some GPs who had not joined the College early on that they felt excluded from the College.

(11) 1983–2002 – International activity

The standing of the College is higher abroad than it is in the UK. Its achievements are recognised internationally and the College has an active programme of fostering international exchanges in all five continents. In the year 2000, the College introduced the MRCGP International examination, yet again it was the first of all the medical Royal Colleges to tailor its examination to the needs of different cultures and countries.

(12) Standards for primary healthcare teams

The Quality Practice Award opened the same technique as the Assessment principles to whole practice teams. No other branch of medicine has yet developed such performance measures.

Leadership training: developing general practice leaders

It is now fashionable for big national organisations to have programmes of leadership training. The College has always functioned as a leadership training organisation, encouraging GPs to take on positions of responsibility in a variety of organisations, and creating many opportunities of its own. It thus has progressively created role models for future generations.

Fifty years on, and at the time of writing, the Chair of the Academy of Medical Royal Colleges, the Chair of the Council of the BMA, the Chair of the Medical Postgraduate Deans, the Director of the London School of Hygiene and Tropical Medicine, the Chief Medical Officer in Scotland, the Chair of the Medical Insurance Agency, the immediate past President of the GMC and the past Chair of the Board of Trustees of Diabetes UK are all or have been GPs. For all these posts, the appointment system or the electoral process is predominantly in the hands of other branches of medicine. All eight of these doctors are FRCGPs.

Some implications for the future

It is important that the College does not rest on its laurels as the challenges general practice faces are no less now than they were 50 years ago. In particular, the College needs to find a solution to two outstanding obstacles: the lack of recognition by the NHS of the MRCGP, so that doctors can still take on unsupervised responsibility in general practice without reaching the College's standard for membership, and secondly the continuing absence of a satisfactory programme of higher professional training in general practice.

Conclusion

In the last 50 years, the organisation of the medical profession has changed greatly. The place of general practice within it has been transformed. Not all of the general practice achievements are due to the College, but more of them are due to the College than any other single organisation, and all of them have been heavily influenced by the College.

In comparison with countries where a college of general practitioners did not develop, or did not develop so early, it is clear that academic development and standard setting has advanced much faster in the UK than in many other countries. Furthermore, on the continent of Europe, it is striking that the countries that have advanced the most, for example the Netherlands, have Colleges of

General Practitioners which are functioning in much the same way as the Royal College of General Practitioners.

The story of the foundation of the second College of General Practitioners in the world, and so the first in Europe, is a story of struggle and achievement. It shows the importance of leadership and planning and how leaders can only succeed if they sense the mood of the times and channel it. It is also a story of challenge and change and, on the whole, remarkable success. British and international general practice and primary care and British medicine generally have all been changed in ways that few could have predicted at the beginning.

The central achievement, which is continuing and which can be celebrated, is releasing the vast range of talent of so many GPs by constant encouragement and empowerment. The key policy for the College has been putting the patients' interests first.

References

1   Cohen Report (1948) *The Training of a Doctor.* Report of the Medical Curriculum Committee of the BMA. Chairman, Sir Henry Cohen. British Medical Association, London.

2   Cohen Report (1950) *General Practice and the Training of the General Practitioner.* Chairman, Sir Henry Cohen. British Medical Association, London.

3   Goodenough Report (1944) Report of the Interdepartmental Committee on Medical Schools. Chairman, Sir William Goodenough. HMSO, Ministry of Health and Department of Health for Scotland.

4   College of General Practitioners (1953) The teaching of general practice by general practitioners. *BMJ.* **2**: 36–8.

5   Curwen M (1964) Lord Moran's ladder. *Journal of the College of General Practitioners.* **7**: 38–43.

6   Pereira Gray DJ (1992) The history of the Royal College of General Practitioners: the first 40 years. *British Journal of General Practice.* **42**: 29–35.

7   Pereira Gray DJ (1992) *Forty Years On: the story of the first forty years of the Royal College of General Practitioners.* Atalink, London.

8   Rose FM and Hunt JH (1951) A College of General Practice [Letter]. *BMJ.* **2**: 1226.

9   Rose FM (1951) Memorandum on the importance of establishing a Royal College of General Practice. *BMJ Supplement 2.* 174–6. [Republished in *Forty Years On: the story of the first forty years of the Royal College of General Practitioners* – see reference no. 7.]

10   Hunt JH (1951) A College of General Practice. *BMJ Supplement.* 174–6.

11   Brain Sir Russell (1952) President of the Royal College of Physicians writing as Chairman of the then three medical Royal Colleges, Letter to the Steering Group. 11 January.

12 McConaghey RMS (1972) Proposals to found a Royal College of General Practitioners in the nineteenth century. *Journal of the Royal College of General Practitioner.* **22**: 775–8.

13 Hunt JH (1973) The Foundation of a College. James Mackenzie Lecture, 1972. *Journal of the Royal College of General Practitioners.* **23**: 5–20.

14 Fry J, Hunt JH and Pinsent RJFH (1963) A *History of the Royal College of General Practitioners: the first 25 years.* MTP, Lancaster.

15 General Practice Steering Committee (1953) A College of General Practitioners Report. Chairman, Sir Henry Willink. *Practitioner.* **170** (Suppl.).

16 Collings JS (1950) General practice in England today: reconnaissance. *Lancet.* **1**: 555–85.

17 Royal College of General Practitioners (1995) *Fellowship by Assessment.* Occasional Paper 50. RCGP, Exeter.

18 Royal College of General Practitioners (1999) *Membership by Assessment of Performance. The MAP Handbook: written guidance for candidates and assessors.* RCGP, London.

19 Royal College of General Practitioners (2000) *Quality in Practice Award.* RCGP, London.

20 Watts CAH (1958) How to compile an age–sex register. *Between Ourselves.* **8**: 1–12.

21 Eimerl TS (1960) Organised curiosity. *Journal of the College of General Practitioners.* **3**: 246–52.

22 Royal College of General Practitioners (1974) *Oral Contraceptives and Health.* Pitman, London.

23 Royal College of General Practitioners (1995) Evidence of the Royal College of General Practitioners to the Select Committee on Science and Technology of the House of Lords. *Medical Research and the NHS Reforms,* HL Paper 12-II, pp. 121–50. HMSO, London.

24 Pereira Gray DJ (1989) The emergence of the discipline of general practice, its literature and the contribution of the College journal. McConaghey Memorial Lecture, 1988. *Journal of the Royal College of General Practitioners.* **39**: 228–33.

25 College of General Practitioners (1965) *Special Vocational Training for General Practice. Report from General Practice No. 1.* CGP, London.

26 Royal College of General Practitioners (1967) *The Implementation of Vocational Training. Report from General Practice No. 6.* RCGP, London.

27 Merrison Committee (1975) Report. Chairman, Sir Alec Merrison. HMSO, London.

28 Royal College of General Practitioners (1995) Table 1. *RCGP Members' Reference Book* 1995b, Appendix 8, p. 94. Camden Publications, London.

29 Pickles WN (1939) *Epidemiology in Country Practice.* Seminal work. The Devonshire Press, Torquay, Devon.

30 Clyne MB (1961) *Night Calls: a study in general practice.* Tavistock, London.

31 Fry J (1961) *The Catarrhal Child.* Butterworth, London.

32 Royal College of General Practitioners (1972) *The Future General Practitioner: learning and teaching.* BMJ Books, London. [Later republished RCGP.]

33 Royal College of General Practitioners (2002) *RCGP Members' Reference Book* 2003: *Fellowship by Assessment.* Campden Publications, London.

CHAPTER 12

Careers: the contribution of women to general practice

Maureen Baker

Women have practised medicine from time immemorial. Aeons before Hippocrates, as priestess, sorceress or wise woman they will have listened, examined and treated those who were fearful, ill or dying. Yet, the history of medicine will record that women were admitted into the medical profession, and then only in very restricted numbers, just over one hundred years ago. From that position, we have now reached a stage where women form the majority of medical school entrants in the United Kingdom, and within ten years, the majority of UK general practitioners will be female. Will this be a threat to general practice, or an opportunity to further enhance our discipline? I believe that women bring a valuable perspective and approach to general practice, just as men do, and that we need, and should celebrate, diversity in our profession on the occasion of the 50th anniversary of the Royal College of General Practitioners.

Women in medicine

The proportion of women in the UK medical workforce has been gradually increasing in the second half of the twentieth century. In 1960, 25% of medical students were women,[1] and this has now risen to over half. The increasing proportion of women joining the medical profession has led to fears that women doctors were being trained at great expense, only to give up work and devote themselves to their families.

These are legitimate concerns, especially when doctors are in short supply, but are they justified? Over the years, various studies have looked at the level of commitment women have demonstrated to their medical careers, and all have found this to be at a surprisingly high level. In 1988, Allen's study of doctors from the 1966, 1976 and 1981 cohorts found that only 5% of women doctors interviewed were not working at all.[2] These findings were reinforced by a later study by the Medical Careers Research Group, which also found a figure of around 5% of women doctors in the cohorts studied were not in paid employment in the UK. According to Allen, 'Comparative studies have indicated that women doctors are more likely than any other group of professional women to continue working when they have family responsibilities and successive studies of women doctors have indicated participation rates of over 90%.'[2]

General practice

The commitment of women doctors to their medical careers has particular implications for general practice due to the high proportion of women in medicine who choose general practice as a career. As fewer male doctors make general practice their first choice of medical career, the influence of women on the discipline increases.

Studies in the early 1980s suggested that women chose general practice for early financial security, the greater flexibility of working practices and because general practice gave women a better opportunity to combine professional and domestic opportunities.[3,4] In their study of four cohorts of doctors who qualified between 1974 and 1983, the Medical Careers Research Group found that with the exception of hours and working conditions – which women rated much more highly as an influence than men – there were no substantial differences between men and women in factors specified as important in making a career choice.[5]

It is therefore not surprising that women doctors had a preference for careers in general practice, in terms of their preferred working practices. However, it is likely that the nature of general practice as a medical discipline is also attractive to women. The new European Definition of General Practice/Family Medicine states:[6]

> General practitioners/family doctors are specialist physicians trained in the principles of the discipline. They are personal doctors, primarily responsible for the provision of comprehensive and continuing care to every individual seeking medical care irrespective of age, sex and illness. They care for individuals in the context of their family, their community and their culture, always respecting the autonomy of their patients. They recognise they will also have a professional responsibility to their community. In negotiating management plans with their patients they integrate physical, psychological, social, cultural and existential factors, utilising the knowledge and trust engendered by repeated contacts. General practitioners/family physicians exercise their professional role by promoting health, preventing disease and providing cure, care or palliation. This is done either directly or through the services of others according to health needs and the resources available within the community they serve, assisting patients where necessary in accessing these services. They must take the responsibility for developing and maintaining their skills, personal balance and values as a basis for effective and safe patient care.

The holistic and nurturing nature of this work, firmly rooted as it is within communities, is in accord with traditional feminine attributes. Our speciality allows men and women to practise a scientific discipline, but in a way that also values human empathy, interaction and warmth.

Our colleagues in hospital medicine also need many of these skills and attributes, but success in hospital medicine has traditionally been based on achievements in research and medical politics. The working practices traditionally followed in these areas are not generally conducive to family life, or indeed to many aspects of life outside medicine, and it is notable that significantly fewer women have opted for this type of career. Nevertheless, there have been some notable exceptions, and their achievements are all the greater for that.

Female medical leadership

Having established that women constitute a significant and increasing section of the medical workforce, it would be interesting to ascertain whether they are able to scale the heights of their profession and attain positions of seniority and responsibility. To many, both lay and medical, the most prized accolade in medicine is the Nobel Prize. Some exceptional women have had the drive and inspiration even to have achieved these heights. Six women have now been awarded the Nobel Prize for Medicine. For the record, and in their honour, they are:

- Gerty Radnitz Cori in 1947, for the discovery of the course of the catalytic conversion of glycogen
- Rosalyn Sussman Yalow in 1977, for the development of radio immuno-assays of peptide hormones
- Barbara McClintock in 1983, for her discovery of mobile genetic elements
- Rita Levi-Montalcini in 1986, for her role in the discoveries of growth factors
- Gertrude Elion in 1988, for her role in the discoveries of important principles of drug treatment
- Christiane Nusslein-Volhard in 1995, for her role in discoveries concerning the genetic control of early embryonic development.

Although no British woman has yet been accorded this accolade, it is generally recognised that Rosalind Franklin played a crucial role in the discovery of the structure of DNA. In 1951, while working under Maurice Wilkins at London's King's College, she took an X-ray photograph of a DNA molecule that was to have a major influence in the subsequent discovery of the double helix structure of DNA. Franklin died of ovarian cancer in 1958 at the age of 37 before Crick, Watson and Wilkins received the Nobel Prize in 1962 for their research (the award is only presented to living candidates).

This illustrates that women can succeed in medicine to the highest level, but for most doctors, awards such as the Nobel Prize barely register on their personal radar. Most of us recognise leadership and success in the championing of special causes, in groundbreaking research or innovation, or in representation. It is important that the young women doctors of today have recognisable role models and champions to whom they can relate. The alternative would be for women in medicine to feel estranged and disenfranchised. This would be deeply regrettable in its own right, but could be frankly dangerous given the emerging gender balance within the profession.

So have we been able to nurture the careers of women doctors in the UK? There is little published evidence in the UK literature. Further afield, a Norwegian study found that men have significantly higher probability for all leadership positions in medicine, and that women are under-represented in higher medical administrative positions. Leadership positions for women were more likely to be found in public health, where working hours are regulated. In hospitals, the proportion of female physicians in the speciality is a determinant for female leadership.[7]

It is not appropriate to generalise from one study in another healthcare system, but can we honestly say that matters are different in the UK? Commenting on the Norwegian findings, the eminent American feminist Elaine Showalter stated that:[8]

> The statistics on leadership and influence in medicine are no different from those in other professions. The picture would look the same if we considered women as deans or chancellors of universities, presidents of corporations, political candidates or film directors. Research and testimony from the professions in general make it clear that sex equality cannot be achieved solely by a focus, however earnest, on the problems of women. The greater challenge is also to change the attitudes of men as well, and to transform public, internalised assumptions that link professional leadership to long hours, sacrifice of personal interests, and stereotypes of managerial style. Women have already overcome many obstacles and accommodated themselves to traditional structures in order to enter a medical profession that long excluded them. If they are to achieve leadership, the profession, as well as the women, will have to change.

These words are a challenge to the entire profession. Given the high and increasing proportion of women in general practice, they are especially challenging for us. How then might we respond to the challenge of supporting women in their general practice careers without disadvantage to male colleagues, and without damaging the very attributes of the discipline that attracted women in the first place?

Future challenges

We need women doctors. In my view, we have always needed them, but at a time when doctors are in short supply in the UK, across Europe and much of the world, then they are an even more precious resource. So we must be able to continue to attract women to medicine and to general practice, and then to retain their skills within the profession.

The desire of many women to combine a worthwhile career with a full and satisfying personal life in terms of having children and raising families will be a major challenge, both for the profession and for those planning the medical workforce. To a certain extent, general practice has adapted to the increasing number of women in the profession and women GPs now have a choice of working patterns: they can work full or part time as GP principals or they can job share. They can choose to work as principals or as locums, deputies, retainers or assistants. The development of Personal Medical Services (PMS) pilots has resulted in significantly increasing the opportunities to work as a salaried doctor in general practice. Many GP principals can choose whether they wish to undertake out-of-hours work as some GP cooperatives, together with deputising services, give doctors the choice whether to delegate their out-of-hours responsibilities to others. Provision of opportunities for flexible working will be one way in which women (and quite possibly an increasing proportion of male doctors) can be attracted to general practice work. But does this mean there will be unacceptable trade-offs? What happens to the hallowed principle of continuity of care, further enshrined in the new European definition of general practice? Can a plethora of female part-timers provide the same continuity that was previously provided in general practice by our male full-time predecessors?

Well, almost certainly not. But that does not mean that the important principles of continuity cannot be enshrined. Patients should normally be able to see the doctor of their choice most of the time. No doctor could ever be expected to be available to their patients for 24 hours every day, 365 days every year. And while patients generally value continuity, they also value choice. It should not be impossible to design systems that will support much continuity of care whilst allowing doctors to have fulfilling personal lives, and patients to choose to see different doctors and health professionals for different problems, within a structure of communication and teamwork.

We also face the very real challenge of having insufficient doctors, including GPs, to meet the demands placed upon the medical workforce. Within the UK, medical student numbers are increasing. But it takes many years to train a doctor, and meanwhile the demand for healthcare provision is also increasing. Almost certainly, new working practices will need to evolve that will allow the best use to be made of the available skills. The case for more critical evaluation of skill-mix is often made clumsily, and in many cases undervalues medical skills, particularly those of the medical generalist. However, it now seems apparent that without significant clinical support for doctors, especially including GPs, many patients could be deprived of the medical and clinical skills necessary for effective healthcare. There are no easy answers when it comes to planning the skill-mix needed to deliver services, but significant developments must be made if we are to safeguard, and hopefully develop, our services to patients.

It therefore becomes imperative that every effort is made to support men and women in remaining within general practice. Doctors of either gender will have career breaks from general practice, or indeed from medicine. Many women doctors will have periods of maternity leave, while both men and women will fall sick from time to time, or travel abroad, or take sabbaticals, or have one of myriad reasons for a period away from general practice. Out in the wider world, it is increasingly the norm for individuals to make frequent career moves: why would we expect GPs to be any different? The days of joining one practice as a young GP and remaining in the practice over the course of a working life are probably long gone for most of us. This is a development unlikely to be controlled, and one which probably brings welcome diversity to working lives. However, it does mean that effective structures need to be in place to ensure that doctors have access to refresher or returner training quickly and with minimum bureaucracy.

To return to the theme of female medical leadership, it will also be important to develop means of supporting those amongst us who have a vision or a passion that might lead to significant developments in the discipline. The flat, non-hierarchical structure of traditional general practice has many strengths: indeed, it may well be of great importance in recruiting doctors into general practice. However, it does lead to difficulties within practices when doctors wish to develop their careers in other areas such as research, medical education, medical management or medico-politics. Such barriers are probably even more insurmountable for many women doctors, given that many have responsibilities for young children at the stages of their careers when they might be ready to explore these avenues. External support is probably necessary for practices to encourage doctors' personal development while still being able to maintain acceptable levels of services for patients.

Conclusion

Women have given much to medicine and to general practice. Many women doctors have led professional lives of quiet service, with dedication and innovation that has often gone unnoticed or uncelebrated. A few have reached positions of distinction and achieved deserved honours and accolades. General practice in particular has benefited from the contributions that all have made. It is fitting to pause and reflect on their achievements at this stage in the development of our discipline, and on the 50th anniversary of the Royal College of General Practitioners. I have no desire or expectation to contribute to the 100th anniversary of the College. I do though have an earnest hope that a similar publication in 2052 will not see any need to devote any particular attention to the achievements of women, just as in this book you will not find a chapter relating to men in medicine. Should that be the case, then I like to think that would indeed be a fitting tribute to women GPs and to women doctors.

References

1 Parkhouse J (1991) *Doctors' Careers: aims and experiences of medical graduates.* Routledge, London.

2 Allen I (1988) *Doctors and their Careers.* Policy Studies Institute, London.

3 Elston MA (1980) Medicine: half our future doctors? In: Silverstone R and Ward A (eds) *Careers of Professional Women,* pp. 99–139. Croom Helm, London.

4 Day P (1982) *Women Doctors: choices and constraints in policies for medical manpower.* King's Fund Centre, London.

5 Lambert T, Goldacre M, Edwards C *et al.* (1996) Career preferences of doctors who qualified in the United Kingdom in 1974, 1977, 1980 and 1983. *BMJ.* **313**: 19–24.

6 European Society of General Practice/Family Medicine (2002) *European Definition of General Practice/Family Medicine.* WONCA, Europe.

7 Kværner KJ, Aasland OG and Botten GS (1999) Female medical leadership: cross-sectional study. *BMJ.* **318**: 91–4.

8 Showalter E (1999) Improving the position of women in medicine. *BMJ.* **318**: 71–2.

CHAPTER 13

Achievements in record keeping: the use of information management and technology

Joe Neary

Much that happens in general practice involves the exchange of information.

In clinical practice, patients communicate their concerns to their general practitioner. These concerns are interpreted by the GP, and securely recorded in notes using medical conventions. The GP communicates information back to the patient, sometimes reinforced by printed information. Prescriptions are relayed (when necessary) to a pharmacist, or a referral may be made to a hospital for an investigation or a specialist opinion. Recorded notes may be used to audit the quality of care, analyse significant events that suggest problems in quality and provide reports in support of patients' financial, social or legal transactions.

This is all so familiar that it may seem banal to restate. But every aspect of this communication has been utterly transformed in the past 50 years. And further changes are rapidly evolving as information is exchanged electronically, and the effects of widespread access to the Internet are felt by patients and professionals alike.

The whole knowledge base of professional practice has been transformed from a stable monolith, reliable for a whole career in medicine, to a rapidly changing, volatile phenomenon. Assumptions about the doctor's greater expertise is ever more likely to be challenged by well-informed patients, undermining previously cherished beliefs about our roles as expert sources of knowledge.

At the time of the College's foundation in the 1950s, clinical notes were brief. Communications with hospitals were fewer. Structured care was undeveloped. Professional knowledge was relatively static and the doctor was always right, even when he (always he!) wasn't. Quality was assumed rather than assured. And computer systems unheard of. Information management was correspondingly rudimentary.

In this chapter, I will outline the changes in information management that have occurred in practice over the past 50 years. Within the limits of a single chapter, the influences on information management cannot be described in full. They are almost co-extensive with all of general practice itself (*see* Box 13.1). Where possible, however, I will relate these changes to the broad pattern of changing demands on general practice.

Box 13.1 Aspects of information management in modern-day general practice

Clinical information
- Maintaining a coherent narrative record
- Communicating with other healthcare professionals:
  - out-of-hours services
  - pharmacists
  - laboratory and X-ray services
  - nursing and other therapists
  - hospital clinics
- Social welfare and insurance
  - benefits and disability
  - insurance claims
  - other civil interests, e.g. driving, legal proceedings
- Use as evidence in the event of complaints or negligence proceedings

Professional knowledge
- Assisted decision making (e.g. Prodigy)
- Education and development (e.g. personal development plans)
- Change management (e.g. implementing defined or revised disease management programmes)
- Research skills (the collection and analysis of research data, critical appraisal)

Quality assurance
- Clinical governance
  - clinical audit
  - risk management (e.g. significant event analysis)
- Appraisal and revalidation portfolios

Practice support
- Financial management (e.g. analysis of financial cash flows)
- Administering NHS claims (e.g. vaccination claims, quality reports from PMS practices)

Starting point

Until recently, the Lloyd George record was the mainstay of clinical records in general practice. These records were famously developed by Lloyd George, then Secretary of State for Social Welfare, to support medical record keeping for workers who were enrolled in the National Health Insurance scheme during the First World War. The size of the record envelopes was dictated by the storage boxes, surplus ammunition boxes of which there was a liberal supply in 1916.

These were fine for primary care up to the 1950s. Hospital correspondence was usually typewritten on flimsy paper sheets which easily folded into the record. GP clinical records were extremely brief. No concept of summarised, formally structured records had been suggested. But as the RCGP commenced a critical examination of general practice from the 1950s onwards, the limitations of the record as it then stood became more apparent.

Through the 1970s, record envelopes became increasingly overloaded with detailed technical information from hospitals. Legal and insurance requests, usually printed on heavy paper, added to the bulk. GPs were observing, diagnosing, treating and recording more on their own account. There was increased recognition of the importance of an adequate record to guide the treatment of the patient, as well as to confirm that effective treatment had been administered. Medical negligence cases began to mount, adding further awareness of the need for detailed note keeping.

A variety of approaches were developed to try to fit an effective record within the constraints of the Lloyd George envelope. Notes were summarised, unnecessary papers stripped out, record envelopes marked in a variety of ingenious ways. All were labour intensive and required an attention to record maintenance bordering on the obsessive.

A4 records

A4 records were suggested as a solution to these increasingly manifest difficulties. First suggested by the RCGP and the GMSC Joint Working Party on the Redesign of Medical Records in General Practice, these were introduced in a haphazard way through the service.

The effective implementation of A4 records required a massive investment in new record storage systems and the administrative time to repack enormous numbers of files. Once effectively introduced, the A4 record resulted in a substantial improvement in the accessibility of the individual record. I remember the pleasure with which I did my first surgery in a practice that had implemented A4 records. The ease with which information could be seen and used was a revelation.

The Department of Health supplied A4 folders and stationery without charge to practices, but they did not make any special provision for the staff and premises investment required to make and sustain the change. Furthermore, when patients moved across practices, records were routinely repacked from A4 to Lloyd George envelopes. These inadequate containers thereby became stuffed more than ever with folded A4 sheets of clinical notes and investigation mounts.

These concerns meant that A4 records were destined to remain a minority 'sport', and were unsustainable in areas with large patient turnover without sacrificial effort.

The demands of audit

A further challenge to record keeping began to arise through the 1980s as the importance of anticipatory care of chronic medical conditions became recognised. This was first fostered by the RCGP through work proposed by John Horder, then President of the College. Its final shape was the 'Quality Initiative' programme, published in 1985.

To carry out such programmes effectively, populations of patients with significant complaints have to be defined. Not only this, but the recommended interventions for these patients have to be recorded in such a way as to allow effective care to be demonstrated. Records have to be systematically and period-ically reviewed to check the effectiveness with which mandated interventions have been carried out, and the intended goals of treatment achieved.

Additional cards were designed and incorporated into records for elderly checks, family planning and a variety of care programmes: diabetes, asthma and hypertension among many others.

The age of clinical audit placed new and unsustainable demands on paper-based records systems. Audit required specific populations of patients to be identified and regularly reviewed.

There were some individuals who managed to maintain the multiple sets of parallel paper records required for these disease registers with commendable effectiveness. The work involved in keeping multiple sets of records to service the needs of programmed care, in addition to the need to maintain an adequate per-sonal record, made this approach untenable for most.

Computerised records

The first shaky steps towards computerisation were taken in the 1970s in Exeter. This relied on the use of large computers which were unaffordable by the mass of GPs. The programming was primitive. Data recording and retrieval required specialist skills. It didn't take off as a general model, though enormously valuable lessons were learned in terms of systems design and the use of computers in support of clinical objectives.

The arrival of cheap and effective microcomputers opened greater possibilities. The Department of Health launched 'Micros for GPs', a limited scheme to foster the uptake of microcomputers by GPs in the early 1980s. These computers were single-user devices with limited data storage and capable of limited functions only. The scheme had very limited funding, was used by few and failed to integrate into daily working routine in most cases.

Then in the mid-1980s, two companies, Vamp (later In-Practice Systems) and Abies (later Meditel, currently Torex), each developed multi-user systems that were capable of supporting a computer terminal on every doctor's desk. These systems were supposed to be financed by the sale of automatically collected information (anonymised) to the pharmaceutical industry.

Now, for the first time, computers could be used to store information relating to patient care at the time of the consultation. And, as payment for the computers was reliant on GPs recording all prescriptions, useful data started to be recorded on computers.

Scotland followed a different route. A single nationally sponsored system, GPASS, was provided free to all Scottish practices from 1990. This system was later to draw criticism due to delays in updating. These delays made the Scottish system appear less developed than the commercially competing systems in England and Wales, though recent developments have overcome many of these problems and GPASS remains by far the dominant system in Scottish general practice.

Coding clinical information

The potential advantages of computers for auditing clinical care were immediately apparent. But then as now, electronic data can only be effectively audited if they are recorded in coded form.

A system for coding comprehensive clinical information was first developed by a Loughborough GP, James Read, in the 1980s. This coding system formed an intrinsic part of the Abies computers, and as it was further developed it was adopted as a national coding system in the early 1990s. It now forms the foundation of medical coding systems used by all of the main computer suppliers in the UK.

As a formal hierarchical set of codes, the Read system doesn't fit comfortably with the ill-defined and multidimensional complaints that often present in general practice. It remains unforgiving in audit if the correct code is not used for key interventions. Blood pressure readings, for example, can only be 'seen' if recorded using the correct code. Various methods are currently in use to try to overcome this limitation, such as the use of formal template systems to enter a structured series of clinical notes.

Further problems with the Read structure of diagnostic coding became immediately apparent when the system was first implemented in hospital environments. These issues could only be addressed by the development of a substantially revised code set, the Read 3 codes. These now run in uneasy parallel with Read 2, which remains the standard for use in the community.

New sets of clinical codes are currently being developed for implementation throughout the UK in the next few years. Called SNOMED-CT (Standard North American Medical Data – Clinical Terms), this system has been developed by the American College of Pathologists with UK participation. It is hoped to overcome many of the problems endemic with the hierarchical and heterogeneous Read codes, though at the time of writing pilot testing has yet to be established, and the expectations await the test of experience.

Many GPs found difficulty in structuring their data records in this way. It adds new and unfamiliar demands to already overstretched consultations. Many practices used their computer systems as simple repeat prescription managers and age–sex registers. Others tried delegating the work of entering more detailed information to practice staff.

It soon became apparent, however, that if computers were going to realise their full potential in auditing the quality of medical care they would have to be used in the consulting room for recording more extensive clinical information. Consultations could not, and still cannot, accommodate the demands of keeping two sets of notes. Either the computer or the paper record was going to suffer.

The 'new contract' of 1991

The new contractual arrangements for general practice implemented in 1991 included new demands for quality assuring general practice. Although these were quite limited in their scope, it was immediately apparent that computers would be important to respond to these new demands. The pill was only slightly sweetened by the provision of 50% subsidies for purchased systems. At this time EMIS emerged, a newcomer to general practice computing that would soon outstrip its longer established competitors.

Further impetus was provided by the arrival of GP fundholding the following year which required highly sophisticated information systems to run the demanding financial management of public funds, and offered more generous reimbursement of computer costs. Not all practices were eligible, or elected, to engage in fundholding, and a disturbing polarisation of practices into 'haves' and 'have nots' subsequently developed, the legacy of which is still apparent.

Fundholding is now a footnote in history, and the 'new contract' of 1991 has now been superseded by a further revision with even more radical implications for practice record systems. Effective information systems in practices are no longer an option. They are essential in delivering the evidence for a multi-dimensional quality framework spanning clinical and administrative standards. Practices that fail to keep pace will be relegated to an economically deprived subclass. The responsibility for paying for enhanced systems, and also the ownership of them, is being transferred to public authorities. These changes will have profound effects on ownership and access to the patient data stored upon them, and this is likely to be a profound source of tension in the future.

The Internet

The Internet has come to maturity as an effective means of communication with over 90% of practices now reportedly connected. This has impacted hugely on clinical applications. Driven prior to 2000 by advances in electronic storage and data analysis, communication protocols have lifted the boundary around practice systems. Many systems now communicate freely with hospital laboratory and radiology services. The futile and labour-intensive business of copying patient notes from computer to paper and back to computer again is being superseded by electronic transfer of records. The physical constraint of the 'practice system' is likely to disappear, as patient records lie in a variety of electronic locations, to be virtually reassembled at the point of each patient contact.

Patients can access enormous information resources easily. In my own practice, this can result in my being presented with disconcertingly thick portfolios of information, some of highly questionable quality, by patients hopeful of unrealistic results from poorly evidenced treatment. It can also help, however, to transform patients from being passive recipients of care to becoming active partners in healthcare; 'co-producers of health' in Julian Tudor Hart's phrase.[1]

With a little skill, the Internet can be used to inform consultations in general practice. Using gateways to quality-assured information patients can be directed to reliable information about their conditions.

Professional development resources have also become more easily available to GPs. A small, but growing, number of universities are offering Internet-based professional education. Most new policy initiatives are fully documented on government websites, notably www.doh.gov.uk/whatsnew. Other useful resources include information on appraisal and revalidation (www.appraisaluk.info and www.revalidationuk.info). A variety of 'portals' (access points that helpfully organise health information) are in development, though none has yet gained dominance. The National electronic Library of Health (www.nelh.nhs.uk/primarycare) is likely to emerge as the brand leader, though the site design remains uninspiring at the time of writing.

Communication is being revolutionised. Instantaneous communication, with exchange of data such as images, text documents, or investigation traces, is now possible. Video links can be incorporated as bandwidth (i.e. the speed with which computers communicate) increases. This means that consultations, even surgical interventions, can be conducted across different continents, though not yet, it seems, between most practices and hospitals in the same neighbourhood in the UK!

When asked, many doctors have expressed more apprehension than enthusiasm to me about the effect of all this information on their practice. The sheer bulk of the information available has a numbing effect. Doctors need to come to terms with the availability of so much information before they can start to interact meaningfully with it.

The new NHS

Since 1997, the direction of development of general practice and, indeed, the whole health service has been explicitly related to the widespread application of information technology.

Standards of healthcare throughout the NHS are to be brought in line with nationally defined standards which reflect opinion on best practice. Standards are to be set, support provided and levels of attainment reviewed and inspected nationally. The most important of the new standards have been published as National Service Frameworks (NSFs) in England and Wales. These are relatively few in number, but wide-ranging in application. To date they cover seven topics, including coronary heart disease, diabetes and mental health. They are also supplemented by a large and rapidly growing number of guidelines issued by the National Institute for Clinical Excellence and its subsidiary collaborating centres.

A detailed health informatics programme has been produced in support of the NSF for Coronary Heart Disease, the first informatics programme in a promised series. This Framework, and the programme, are built on a number of important assumptions.

First, the new information that is enshrined in the NSF must be sufficiently familiar to doctors and other professionals to ensure commitment to implement it. In fact, much of this information has been widely publicised, but there may still be gaps in the knowledge of some clinicians. Support will be needed for making the appropriate changes in practice, and change management skills to ensure that the changes occur and their uptake is evaluated.

Second, the interventions mandated in the NSF will be effectively conducted in general practice consultations. To help to achieve this, clinical templates have been developed for the leading general practice systems. These add-ons sometimes interrupt the flow of the consultation, however. It can be difficult to use them when the patient's main concerns may be on complex psychosocial issues distantly related to their heart disease. Consultation times may need to be considerably longer than their current nine-minute average to allow such extensions to the clinical agenda.

Third, the information that demonstrates successful completion of these protocols will be analysed and reported. In some cases, the information required may need to be drawn from a number of different sources and may be used for audit and benchmarking. Strict measures to preserve patient confidentiality are essential.

Fourth, the comprehensive evidence specified by new quality frameworks has confirmed the importance of fully computerised medical records for delivery. The move to 'paper-light' or 'paperless' practice has now evolved from innovation to full-scale adoption. It is likely that the great majority of practices will rely on computers as their primary clinical records system by the end of this decade.

The issues concerned were recognised by the RCGP's Health Informatics Group in the 1990s. They published detailed specifications for quality and security in keeping electronic patient records in 2000.[2]

Modernising the health service

The NSFs are just one item in an increasingly ambitious agenda to modernise the English health service (there are corollaries to these frameworks in other parts of the UK). Extended use of electronic information is fundamental to many of these agendas.

In this vision, patients will be cared for by a diverse range of professionals in the community and in hospitals. Traditional professional roles will be over-ridden by the imperative to ensure that the service provided to the patient is delivered efficiently and effectively. In practical terms, this requires ever larger groups of people to have access to the whole, or a substantial part, of personal health records.

Communications between primary care and hospitals are expected to become streamlined. Once again, electronic clinical details will be at the heart. GPs will be able to access hospital appointments, as well as laboratory and imaging information. Part of their records will need to be accessible in turn to hospital services. Clinical information will be transmitted instantly across electronic networks at a touch of the proverbial button. In practice this vision has faced a succession of thorny problems, and effective communication across the community–hospital divide is some years behind schedule.

In the most evolved current vision, the health record will no longer be based on a single deposit of information on an isolated site, but will draw, as the need arises, from different items stored on different systems and brought together in a location to serve the needs of that consultation or enquiry. So analysis of clinical quality can occur at locations distant from the consultation record. And patients will no longer be limited to being seen in the one location where their physical health record is situated. Storage of general practice records in super-servers in the primary care organisation is beginning to emerge in some areas.

This trend may accelerate as new investment in primary care informatics is made at the behest of primary care organisations in the wake of the 2003 contract.

Information tensions in the modernisation agenda

Current government policies appear to help to address the concerns about uneven implementation of best practice, first articulated by Archie Cochrane in 1971.[3] Evidence on best practice on the most important health problems is being defined and collated. It is being enshrined in practice, with considerable incentives on offer. Evidence is being sought for their effective implementation. So organisations concerned with quality in healthcare, such as the RCGP, should be delighted. Many of the College's long-held ambitions appear to be on the verge of fulfilment.

But in fact, concerns have been growing. It is these concerns that will shape the future development of information management in general practice.

Security in data management

Ever wider access to patient information, storage of data in locations outside the control of the responsible clinician, the capacity to distribute sensitive information to a large readership at the touch of a button – all of these are issues that challenge our current standards on privacy. The disquieting occasions on which patients express concern about their clinical information, or ask me not to record potentially important information in their record, are becoming more numerous.

The arguments concerning access to records are subtle. Not all records warrant the same treatment. Patients might understandably want the fact and circumstances of an HIV test kept entirely private between themselves and their own doctor. On the other hand, they might well want their allergy to penicillin or the fact that they are taking warfarin easily available to a wide circle of clinicians. With the changes in out-of-hours arrangements, greater numbers of vulnerable and ill patients are being managed in the community by an increasing diversity of clinicians. These issues will continue to surface.

Security in communication

Within the next few years, clinical records are due to be transferred electronically as patients move between practices. Hospitals and practices will exchange information electronically; providing mutual access for practices and hospitals to each other's clinical records across the NHS net has been mooted. Pressure will rise for greater access to records from other appropriate bodies.

Any exchange of patient-identifiable information across electronic networks may be hazardous. These hazards cannot be entirely avoided with current technology. They can be substantially reduced by ensuring that the sender of every message from a clinical system can be accurately identified by a coded tag. These tags are the electronic equivalent of a signature. All clinical information must be encrypted when going through a network. Modern encryption is highly sophisticated. Messages and documents can easily be made indecipherable other than by their intended recipients.

If systems are properly designed, security can in many ways be greater than in the exchange of paper records. Ensuring that this is so involves technical issues that are highly complex, analysed and discussed in rarefied terms and impenetrable to the uninitiated.

Understanding the problems of electronic communications sometimes requires expert review. The RCGP, along with the BMA and the Primary Care Specialist Group of the British Computer Society, has sponsored a dedicated group of GP health informaticians since the mid-1990s. This group keeps current and proposed information policy under close review. It analyses the underlying technical issues in depth.

Training and development

The training and development agenda for information management is immense. Currently, the emphasis is on acquiring simple computer skills in the form of the European Computer Driving Licence (ECDL), and the consistent use of clinical terms. As the use of computers in consultations becomes more widespread, and especially as doctors learn to type as fast as they currently (and far less legibly) write, much of the mystique around computers will dissipate.

These are arguably the easiest of the challenges that confront GPs. More troubling is the change in social attitudes towards professional knowledge and expertise. Our knowledge base is no longer discrete, stable or the privileged prerogative of doctors alone.

Rapidly evolving medical evidence has meant that knowledge is time-limited. As interventions become more effective and as their risks increase, the contrast between the outcomes of good quality and poor quality care are ever more clearly visible. Education and training to deal with these challenges is neither easy nor cheap. Current practice resources are wholly inadequate to the task. Knowledge and quality management on this scale can only be delivered following a step change in the support available to practices.

References

1 Tudor Hart J (1988) *A New Kind of Doctor.* Merlin Press, London.

2 Joint Computing Group of the General Practitioners' Committee and the Royal College of General Practitioners (2000) *Good Practice Guidelines for General Practice Electronic Patient Records.* General Practitioners' Committee and the RCGP, London.

3 Cochrane AL (1971) *Effectiveness and Efficiency.* Nuffield Provincial Hospitals Trust, London.

Further reading

Feldbaum EG and Dick RS (1997) *Electronic Patient Records, Smart Cards and Confidentiality. Financial Times,* London.

Lervy B (1996) *Medical Records in Practice.* Practice Organisation Series 2. Royal College of General Practitioners, London.

NHS Executive (1998) *Information for Health: an information strategy for the modern NHS 1995–2005.* Department of Health Publications, Wetherby. www.doh.gov.uk/ipu/strategy. index.htm

Preece J (2000) *The Use of Computers in General Practice.* Churchill Livingstone, London.

Pringle M, Dixon P, Carr-Hill R *et al.* (1995) *Influences on Computer Use in General Practice.* Occasional Paper 68. Royal College of General Practitioners, London.

CHAPTER 14

The future of general practice

David Haslam

The more everything changes, the more it stays the same.

Most quotations about the future tend to be depressingly negative, or embarrassingly inaccurate, but this apparently simple thought is perhaps one of the most positive because the only other thing that we know about our predictions is that they will inevitably be wrong.

Following the RCGP's 50th anniversary year, it is only right that we should also look forward to our next 50 years. But it is with a sinking heart that I realise that this chapter, appearing in a book that will sit in medical libraries for many years and which could be pored over by historians in the future, is likely to cause more amusement in the years to come than anything else in the book. Life can only be lived forwards, and understood backwards, and yet I am here attempting to peer into the future and make my predictions.

After all, look at some of the great predictions that have been oft quoted from the past. Charles Duvall of the US Patents Office said in 1899 that 'everything that can be invented has been invented'. In 1895, Thomas Edison was equally far-sighted with his memorable phrase that 'the possibilities of the aeroplane have been exhausted', and in 1948 the Annual Report for IBM stated quite categorically that 'the computer has no commercial future'. The only thing that we cannot predict with any clarity is the future.

But general practice certainly has a future. It may change, it may develop, it may strengthen, but it will survive. After all, it is a quite astonishingly successful branch of medicine, delivering eight out of ten patient contacts within the NHS, with approximately one million consultations every single day in 2002. It enjoys higher satisfaction ratings that almost any other public service.[1] For year upon year patients in the UK have seen their general practitioner as an advocate, as a friend, as a locally available expert and as an essential part of their community.

But this does not mean that general practice has been stagnant. Fifty years ago most care was delivered by one or two doctors, probably practising in their own homes, with a team that consisted of the doctor's wife and remarkably little in the way of support staff or equipment or even genuinely effective medication.

Today, GPs typically work in group practices with a group of other doctors and a primary healthcare team that would have been seen as beyond the wildest dreams of the doctor from 50 years ago.

Yet, with all these changes, the core role of the GP has not changed. The most important moments in healthcare occur in the privacy of the consulting room, after the patient has come in and closed the door. This personal relationship should not have changed over the last 50 years, and must not change in the future. If we were to lose the security and safety of the consulting room, the personal caring touch or the doctor who knows the patient as a person, it would be a disaster for our society.

Nevertheless, despite all these strengths and the high esteem in which general practice is held, all is not well in the state of general practice. The external world is changing faster than anyone would have predicted: there are major workforce shortages both in medicine and in nursing, increasing patient expectations, increasing demand for accountability by government and a rapidly and significantly changing demographic structure of our society. In addition, the new genetics will have a major effect on the way that all doctors, including GPs, work. Indeed, if there is one area in which we can barely predict how the future will turn out, it must be genetics. In the same way that even current developments in Internet technology were barely dreamed of 20 years ago, so is genetic science almost entirely unpredictable. If GPs try to continue working over the next 50 years as they do at present, the system will not survive. Nor will it deserve to survive. It is therefore vital that we change and evolve, whilst at all times retaining those things that are most important and most valued by our patients.

Perhaps the main change that is facing the medical profession relates to the extraordinary and rapid rise of the availability of information on the Internet. Barely predicted only a few years ago, the Internet has fundamentally changed the relationships between all professions and their lay publics. In the past, a profession could be defined by the body of knowledge that it held. Professor Sir George Alberti, as President of the Royal College of Physicians, often described the arrival of information technology as being similar to the translation of the Bible from Latin. When the Bible was only available in the Latin language, the priest controlled all access to this knowledge. Translation of the Bible freed up this access, changing entirely the role and position of the clergy for their congregations, and for society as a whole.

A similar seismic shift has affected our congregations. On a computer with an Internet connection, currently costing less than £500, any of our patients can now access almost all the medical knowledge in the world. Doctors no longer control this knowledge. There are those who find this deeply uncomfortable, but resisting this development is as futile as King Canute resisting the tide.

Case history
A patient wrote to me a few days before his consultation. With his letter he enclosed the printouts of two papers, one from the *Lancet* and one from the *New England Journal*

of Medicine, that he had found on the Internet. These related to possible treatments for his cancer. In his accompanying letter he said that he thought I might like to read these before the consultation. When he subsequently consulted me he asked me what I thought. I explained that I felt somewhat out of my depth with some of the technical descriptions in the papers, and that I wanted him to realise that I was not an expert in prostate cancer, and that I was almost certainly not the right person to advise him. He needed to talk to his urologist about all this. He looked at me and smiled. 'I know you're not an expert in prostate cancer,' he said, 'but you are an expert in me.'

The role of the GP in the future will be much less involved in imparting knowledge, and far more involved in sharing understanding of that knowledge, guiding, mentoring and being the patient's advocate through the complexities of the healthcare system. This will inevitably change our role, but in no way will it diminish it. After all, it is not our health that is at issue, it is the patient's health.

Training

So how will the GP appear in the future? What will their training, career structure and working day be like? In recent years, it has become increasingly clear that current training for general practice is far from adequate for the complexity of the task. Currently, fledgling GPs have only three years of postgraduate vocational training, of which two years are spent in secondary care specialities. There is almost no logic to this arrangement. The training for a speciality should be based within that speciality. There is no doubt that secondary care can teach the young GP many skills that will be invaluable in their future careers, but the focus of their training should, and must, be based in general practice.

It should also become expected, rather than simply desirable, that all new GPs should have passed the MRCGP examination. For decades it has been expected that all surgeons would have passed the FRCS, and all hospital physicians would have passed the MRCP. What possible logic can there be for accepting lower standards in the speciality in which doctors practise almost always unsupervised, are frequently isolated, and make some of the most difficult front-line decisions?

Following the end of vocational training, all doctors would then benefit from a spell of higher professional education, continuing with the group support and mentorship that proves so valuable through the training years. At present, at the moment when most support is needed – at the start of a doctor's career – it generally fades away, leaving doctors both isolated and in a position to begin to make the same mistakes with ever increasing confidence.

After passing the MRCGP examination, and joining the Royal College, all doctors already have an obligation both to keep up to date and to demonstrate their competence through revalidation. The RCGP is continuing to develop a Professional Development scheme that offers support and mentorship for GPs, as well as guiding them into firstly uncovering and then addressing their learning needs. In years to come, one might hope and expect that all GPs would avail themselves of such a scheme which helps to educate, support and encourage as well as dealing with revalidation, appraisal and clinical governance.

As part of a doctor's professional development, whether through the Accredited Professional Development (APD) scheme or not, it will be completely essential that the doctor has protected time within the working week for education, audit, research and mentoring activities. At the moment such a concept is but a dream, but it is a dream with powerful friends,[2] and is essential if the profession is to survive and thrive.

Career development

Research has shown that burn-out and stress tend to be significantly less in doctors who do not work full time in the front line as GPs.[3] The development of special medical interests, in which part of the doctor's working week will be focused on an area different from their front-line care, would almost certainly carry the same benefits in terms of protection of enthusiasm and prevention of burn-out. When the workforce allows, and at present the workforce pressures are a major stumbling block for all these developments, it would be an ideal aspiration for every GP to become a GP with a special interest. These special interests need not be just clinical. Whilst clinical activities such as GPs with special interests in dermatology, endoscopy and rheumatology, among many others, are valuable both for patients, the doctor and the NHS, there are many other areas in which GPs with special interests can carry out work of significance and importance.

For years GP trainers have simply been GPs with a special interest in education. GPs with a special interest in research should have the time and expertise acknowledged and resourced. GPs with special interests in mentorship and service development should similarly benefit their colleagues and the NHS. To develop special expertise will inevitably protect and prolong a doctor's career, helping to maintain enthusiasm.

Indeed, if we look far enough and optimistically enough into the future, it is possible to see a vision in which many, if not most, GPs continue to develop their careers throughout their working lives. For far too long, general practice has had no career structure, unless the doctor invents it for themselves. It has been possible to do the same job, at the same desk, with the same patients for over 35 years. For some, this is enough. For most, it is a recipe for burn-out and disillusionment.

Interest and expertise in areas of special interest may lead to the development of diplomas, to provide evidence of such expertise. In time, these diplomas could take the form of credits towards higher degrees. Already, significant numbers of doctors are taking Master of Science (MSc) courses and other higher qualifications. If workforce pressures, time, funding and mentorship are available then there is no reason why the majority of GPs should not choose this route. Currently, such a belief may seem almost laughable. I hope that in 50 years these words will be read with complete incredulity that this was ever not the norm.

In addition, it is clearly logical that this education activity, taken at the doctor's own pace and responding to the doctor's educational needs and interests, with protected supported time, will link into the RCGP's quality award system such as Fellowship by Assessment and the Quality Practice Award. Whilst such schemes may appear overwhelming to many doctors today, if they are treated like an elephant sandwich and tackled bit by bit in a go-your-own-pace modular methodology, they will be seen as an aspiration that anyone can achieve. Indeed, perhaps one day every GP will aspire to Fellowship by Assessment at some stage in their career.

Writing these words at a time of a major workforce crisis and desperately low morale in general practice, I am all too well aware that these aspirations may seem unrealistic. At the same time, Britain's GPs are extraordinarily enthusiastic, altruistic and positive – when they are supported. Support has been sadly lacking within the NHS, but if career development and educational aspiration can be built into the system then the sky is, indeed, the limit. At the present time the NHS recruits altruistic young people, fails to support them and then wonders where their altruism went. We all have the opportunity to correct this.

Patients

What of the patients? Recent reports such as the Wanless Report[4] into the National Health Service and the report from the BMA think tank[5] have suggested that the great majority of the front-line work of primary care can, and should, be carried out by nurses, leaving doctors to concentrate on apparently more complex cases. This fundamentally fails to appreciate the complexity of the task carried out by GPs. Because it looks easy, it doesn't mean that it is.

Whilst much front-line work can be carried out by nurses and nurse practitioners, and indeed will logically also be carried out by other team members such as pharmacists and physiotherapists, there is nevertheless a great range of undifferentiated initial presentations that pose as great a challenge as any faced by any doctor in any speciality. Unravelling the complexity of a headache can be a major task, with causes from the purely physical to the purely psychological, with every conceivable station in between.

So the choice as to who is consulted must remain with the patient. They must not be coerced into automatically seeing a nurse first, any more than every case needs to see a doctor first. Patients must be able to choose whom they see. They may choose to see a doctor, a nurse practitioner, a nurse or indeed any other primary care therapist, but the choice must be theirs. GPs will still have a very clear role in the front line of the NHS. It is often poorly recognised that general practice functions as the 'risk sink' for the NHS, in the same way that mechanical and electronic machines often require 'heat sinks'. Without the ability to absorb and deal with risk and uncertainty, referral and investigation rates would increase dramatically, almost certainly leaving the NHS as an unviable organisation. The secret to effective front-line care is patient-centred skill mix, with each practitioner having adequate time to perform their tasks.

There can also be no doubt that personal continuity of care will be just as important in the future as it is today. Although a great deal of future medical care will be team based, and information technology and smart cards will allow sharing of information and results, people need people. Individual patients will develop working relationships with individual doctors whom they feel they can trust. They always have and they always will, and it is vital that any structuring of healthcare in the years to come allows for this. The more complex life becomes, the more does the simple caring human interaction matter.

The structure and organisation of general practice in the next few years is likely to become almost unrecognisable. But the single most important activity in any doctor's work will remain as important as ever. The consultation – that private and intensely personal relationship between two people – is an activity that has spanned the centuries. For all the changes of technology, of teamworking and skill-mix, or of new therapies and diagnostic techniques, the one-to-one doctor–patient relationship must remain the centre of the medical universe. Indeed, in an increasingly depersonalised and technological world, the intimacy of caring and understanding will become increasingly important.

The more complicated the world becomes, the more the GP will be needed. There are few professional groups that can be more certain that they have a future, but it is one we need to embrace with open minds. As the American social philosopher Eric Hoffer once said, 'In a time of drastic change it is the learners who inhabit the future. The learned usually find themselves equipped to live in a world that no longer exists.' Be warned, and enjoy the journey. If we retain our core values, then we can be optimistic rather than fearful. The book that is published for the RCGP's 100th anniversary will certainly make for fascinating reading.

Case history
It is July 2052. Simon Bartlett enters his GP's consulting room. Holding his thumb against the touch-sensitive pad on the doctor's desk for a few seconds results in his full and updated, international medical record being displayed on the visual display unit built into the doctor's workstation. Laura Stansfield has been Simon's family doctor for several years now. Working in a team of NHS therapists, whose modular inter-professional training has led to great appreciation of each other's strengths and potential, Laura prides herself on her personal holistic approach. A voice recognition system

records the whole consultation, producing key words for the summary. Simon's medication, which requires lipid lowering, hypotensive and diabetes treatments, is combined in a single, bespoke, once-daily tablet, formulated to his exact personal needs. The visual display unit displays the daily blood pressures that have automatically been recorded since his last consultation. Some fine-tuning of his medication is required, advised by the auto-pharmacy advisor. But then he says, 'While I'm here doctor, it's my wife. I'm so worried about her.' And the tears begin to flow ...

References

1   NHS Executive (1999) *National Survey of NHS Patients*. NHSE, Leeds.

2   Wanless D (2002) *Securing our Future Health: taking a long-term view*. HM Treasury, London. www.hm-treasury.gov.uk/wanless

3   Kirwan M and Armstrong D (1995) Investigation of burn-out in a sample of British general practitioners. *British Journal of General Practice*. **45** (394): 259–60.

4   Wanless D (2002) *Securing our Future Health: Taking a long term view*. Final report. HM Treasury, London.

5   British Medical Association (2002) *A New Model for NHS Care*. BMA, London.

CHAPTER 15

The general practitioner and the spirits of time

Per Fugelli

Peripatetic lecture to celebrate the 50th anniversary of the Royal College of General Practitioners in Edinburgh, Perth, Glasgow, Aberdeen and Inverness.

Thirty years ago I worked as a young general practitioner on an Arctic island 100 kilometres west of the Norwegian mainland, in good company with my wife, my son and 2000 wild and wise natives. However, from a medical point of view, I was on a lonely planet. The nearest colleague was located 50 kilometres away with a frenetic maelstrom between us. There was no general practice pride or College in Norway in those times – indeed the medical establishment regarded GPs as underdogs. But I felt like a lion on my island. I loved my work, experiencing every day loaded with intellectual delight, practical utility and the joy of human encounters. My pons cerebri harboured a conviction of general practice as a speciality in its own right, with its own elementary particles, its own specific gravity. I knew this as a tacit instinct. I lacked words, concepts, definitions and a structure: a paradigm.

Then, in 1972, a book landed on my island: *The Future General Practitioner*.[1] This RCGP publication acted as an intellectual lift. Suddenly a basic instinct was transformed to rational evidence: my professional solitude was replaced by a community spirit and I joined the bandwagon of general practice, coached by the RCGP. I will always be indebted to the College for rescuing my GP identity on that lonely planet in 1972.

The Kalahari inspiration

When, in an act of vanity I accepted the invitation to give this demanding lecture, I fled in panic to the Kalahari Desert of Botswana, hunting and gathering inspiration among the Basarwa, the bushmen. Here is what I found.[2,3]

The Royal College of Traditional Healers

The healers of the Kalahari are general practitioners *par excellence*. They are what you are in ultimate crystallisation: masters of personal doctoring, genuine generalists, near-life doctors, in-society doctors. They are soulmates with their patients. They belong to the very same flock. They share history, destiny and future.

The ancestors' spirits

The healers are online with their ancestors' spirits. According to the healers, disease is not a phenomenon *per se*, as claimed by Western biomedical superstition. Disease is nothing but a symptom, signalling the wrath of the ancestors. Disease is vengeance, and the avengers are demons.

The demons

They will haunt you, induce pain, create fever and even kill your body if peace with the ancestral spirits, the guardians of eternal values, is not restored. Therefore the targets of the healer's intervention in the Kalahari are not molecules but sins, not cells but souls, not individuals but social ecosystems. The healer's challenge is to diagnose the broken values, exorcise the demons and guide the perplexed into a new and better life. Their technique is 'boiling energy'.[4]

The healing dance

The healing dance takes place at night around the fire. A flock of between 10 and 40 Basarwa participate in hours of monotonous, suggestive clapping, singing and dancing. They accumulate sufficient energy for the healer to enter into a trance. The trance is introduced by a shriek and convulsions. During the trance, the healer passes over to The Other Side, where he consults with the ancestors' spirits. Awakened by central nervous system-stimulating vapours from a turtle-shield, he comes back to the patient's life world with a prescription for hope.

Demonology at home

In this lecture I will use the technique of the Kalahari healers. I will dance with the general practitioners of Scotland, fall into a trance, consult with the ancestral and live spirits of the Royal College of General Practitioners,[5–9] diagnose and exorcise:

- demons in the doctors' minds
- demons and angels in the souls of our patients
- demons in the Scottish domain.

A strange analogy, you may feel, and reject my attempt to apply a 30 000-year-old Kalahari explanatory model on modern Scotland and post-modern medicine AD 2002. You may be right. It is a wild, culture transplantation experiment, but I have three arguments to suppress your intellectual immune system.

We are of the same basic stock

Humans are humans, healers are healers, be it in the thirst lands of Botswana or the Highlands of Scotland. When we disclose the local cultural masquerade, see through our fancy dresses – be it the Bushman's loincloth or the Scotsman's kilt – the naked man is a truly globalised creation.

Another reason for accepting demonology at home may be derived from this equation:

$$m = b \times c \times p^2$$

which postulates that medicine = biology × culture × politics squared.

Medicine is inclined to believe that it is alone in the world, and that clinical practice can be performed in a scientific heaven isolated from earthly contamination – but that is not so. The medical profession is inclined to believe that it is a rational body of autonomous men and women who practise medicine unconfounded by passions and fashions, follies and fallacies, angels and demons – but it is not so. No patient is an island. No doctor is an alien. What happens in the microcosm of the consultation is a reflection of what goes on in the macrocosm of society. Hopes, expectations and complaints expressed in our surgeries echo the collective soul of modern times. So it is in the Kalahari, and so it is in Scotland.

Scutte

Are Scots and Basarwa more equal than other people? When the Roman legions invaded Scotland 1900 years ago, they were forced to retreat and hide behind Hadrian's Wall. The Romans were conquered by a strong and wild people they named Scutte, which in Latin means 'the wandering nation'. You were nomads wandering in the mountains and valleys, searching like the Bushmen of the Kalahari for food, water, shelter, dignity and love. And like the Basarwa, you love your land – the birthplace of valour, the country of worth. You, like the Basarwa, sing:[10]

> My heart's in the Highlands, my heart is not here
> My heart's in the Highlands, a chasing the deer.

I have now tested the cultural compatibility between Kalahari and Scotland and found it satisfactory. You are indeed closely related, so transplantation may be feasible. Therefore it makes sense to chase demons not only in the heart of Africa, but also in the minds of modern doctors and in the soul of Cool Britannia.

In the spiritual mirage of the Kalahari, we are incited to ask:

- Can modern patients be possessed?
- Who are the wizards of medicine and society today?
- Who are the healers of modern times?

So let us borrow the conceptual bow and the analytical arrow of the Bushman, and go out in the post-modern jungle hunting for demons. And why not start with 'the enemy within', under the motto 'Doctor heal thyself'?

Demons in the minds of the doctors

Modern medicine is possessed by demons.

The demon of scientism

The general practitioner and writer William Carlos Williams said: 'But the whole world has been and is blinded now by the effects of science and philosophy from birth up. Science is a deceit; philosophy a sham; these are not life, but a scum over it through which we see torturedly. But poetry [he means general practice] is the breath of life itself.'[11]

There is now an urge worldwide for more research, documentation, quality control and evidence-based standards in clinical medicine. I see a danger of scientific overkill, with devaluation of clinical judgement and personal wisdom. Theodore Fox, former editor of the *Lancet*, claimed: 'The patient may well be safer with a physician who is naturally wise, than with one who is artificially learned.'[12] The GP is the streetwise guy of medicine. Scientism must not be the one and only true love for the practitioner. We must revalue practical wisdom as used by each one of you in the consultation room and acknowledge that the healing dance can never be evidence based.

The demon of 'too-muchness'

The next demon tormenting medicine is 'too-muchness'. Modern medicine promises people too much certainty, too much healing, too much prevention.[13,14] Researchers, specialists and public health doctors emerge as the new Almighty, heralding zero-vision: invest billions in our brains and laboratories and we shall give you Heaven on Earth, with zero risk, zero suffering, zero disease and zero death. The burden of perfection makes doctors sink with exhaustion. The megalomaniacal promises make patients sink with frustration. The RCGP should produce a placard to hang prominently in all consulting rooms:

> We must accept our pain, change what we can, and laugh at the rest.
>
> Camille Paglia

We should promote a health education which cures people from having unrealistic expectations, confesses the ignorance of medicine and admits the uncertainty of clinical practice. Each one of us can do so in the consultation, but in addition concerted, collective efforts are necessary. Perhaps the RCGP should also establish a GP fire brigade that flies out to the public to extinguish false hopes and real fright ignited by mad-cow specialists and speculative media.

The demon of 'too-muchness' has a Siamese twin called the demon of medical inflation.

The demon of medical inflation

Modern techno-medicine converts more and more common risks, biological variation, natural stress and life's own troubles into diagnoses which demand specialised investigation and therapy.[13,15] The result may be learned helplessness among patients. The doctor will also be in trouble on Medication Island. He will lose professional identity, be a master of none. Society will suffer too as healthcare costs explode. The tonnage of trifles and banalities may displace essential needs. What to do? The RCGP should produce one more placard to hang prominently in all consulting rooms:

> I am not in this world to fulfill your expectations.
>
> Saul Bellow

We must abandon our eager-to-please mentality and restore the noble art of saying 'No'.

The Prince of Darkness

Doctors work on the dark side of life. That may obscure our minds. We become obsessed by anomalies, failures, dangers, suffering, disabilities and death.[16] In

Machiavelli's textbook, *The Prince*,[17] there is a chapter on how to stay in power by creating fear and then offering protection. Modern doctors are like medical princes of darkness, promoting risk instead of trust, prescribing epidemiological verdicts instead of faith, catalysing surrender instead of fight. To use a metaphor: 'Thou flyest to thy cave of sorrow' instead of 'Joy returned to the hill of hinds'.[18]

Our colleagues in the Royal College of Traditional Healers in the Kalahari are medical princes of light and hope. They vitalise the doctor within the patient. And sometimes they blow up the very Cochrane base with the nuclear power that resides in human souls.

The GP works close to life. He observes the dark sides, but also the bright sides in The Book of Man. Therefore GPs are qualified to dethrone the medical Prince of Darkness and install a doctor who can guide the patients from the cave of sorrow to the hill of hinds.[18]

Healing in the House of Medicine

The GP translates medicine to people's life world. This should be reversed; we must translate people's life world to medicine, too. We must help our autistic colleagues in the House of Medicine to communicate with life and reality. Many of the powers in medicine, be it in academic medicine or in health policy, reside on distant planets. They execute high-impact medicine far from peoples' lives in Edinburgh on a Monday. Medicine designed on distant planets may not work on Earth. Highbrow medicine may even be dangerous to people in the Lowlands.[13,15] Therefore medicine needs GPs as mediators of realism, conveyors of common sense and as storytellers of a day in the life of 'John Smith'. We should act more courageously as messengers of grounded, clinical experiences to the spin-doctors at the top of the medical hierarchies. We must help medicine to develop a 'people-centred method', ensuring communication with the folk-soul and compatibility with the facts and mysteries of life.

Demons in the minds of the patients

The demons infesting the House of Medicine are those of scientism, 'too-muchness', medical inflation and the Prince of Darkness. But demons are not permanent residents – evil spirits wander. They migrate from the souls of doctors to the minds of patients. Here they rise again in the guise of the following.

The demon of healthism

There is a strong imperative for health in contemporary society.[15] People strive for perfect health because it has become the key to happiness. However, the modern health cult is a delusion opposing biological laws, contradicting life itself. The imperative for health produces stress, disease and extravagant demands on healthcare.

The strait-jacket of health also steals freedom from people and society. I have a presentiment of a medico-moralistic police state silently emerging, hidden behind the holy mantra: health. A foreboding of a brave new Scotland where gene-technicians, psychomolecule-designers and social engineers lead every citizen into a state of complete physical, mental and social well-being.

Modern times require that the GP counteracts healthism. The GP works with misery and happiness, beauty and ugliness, wickedness and goodness. The GP understands that imperfection is the lot of man and that a sound health culture includes unavoidable pain, trouble and malfunction. The GP can advocate the human right to be imperfect.

The demon of discontent

Scientism is converted in the patient to healthism. Medicine's second demon, 'too-muchness', rises again in the patient as discontent. Fascinated by zero-vision, people will not see the limitations of medicine. Enchanted by heavenly expectations they will not tolerate earthly realities. When the spell is broken, they experience disease as a violation of rights, a sober 'no' as an insult and death as a capital punishment, which is converted to complaints, grievances, claims of compensation and action for damages. Medicine becomes the Wailing Wall instead of the Well of Comfort and Reward.

Can the GP belittle the demon of discontent? Yes, by three means.

Firstly, by emphasising that nature not medicine is the only superpower, and by admitting and even marketing the limits of man-made medicine. Secondly, by reinstating sound fatalism into the soul of the people.

The third remedy against the demon of discontent may be controversial. We ought to reprimand unreasonable and demanding patients, tell them how spoilt they are, and even say 'Shame on you'. We ought to remind them of the fact that in Eritrea there are three doctors per 100 000 inhabitants. In Mali, the public health expenditure is £12 per inhabitant per year. In Zambia, people desperate from hunger dive into crocodile-infested rivers, searching for edible plants and roots. We should recommend that our patients sing hymns of praise to Aneurin Bevan, to God, to the oil in the North Sea, to their doctors, who make them the most privileged people on Earth.

The demon of fear

Medicine's Prince of Darkness reflects in the patient as the demon of fear. If we fly to the moon and look down on the world, if we travel with a time-machine and look back on history, there can be no doubt that people in Scotland live in the safest place on Earth, in the safest second in history. We are uniquely secure in our societies, protected from the classic inflictions of mankind: pestilence, hunger, poverty and war. But nevertheless our suprarenal glands are on red alert.[19] We fear mad cows, carcinogenic strawberries, mobile phones softly boiling our brains, vaccines imprisoning our children in autism, doctors operating as silent killers. The GP can act as a tranquilliser, contradicting the apocalyptic prophesies from double-blinkered epidemiologists, extraterrestrial researchers and the dramatising media. The GP can arrest the adrenaline pushers by interpreting the new in the light of the old, and by moderating the piece in the context of the whole.

Healing in the consulting room

The consultation may in some respects be regarded as a spiritualistic séance. Not that the GP roles his eyes and shrieks, but our practice creates spirits, expectations and addictions in the patient. GPs do mould people's health and illness culture by their sheer being, by their pure doing. Each of you will have 140 000 to 160 000 patient encounters during your professional lifetime. This year 25 million direct patient contacts will occur in Scottish general practice. This provides the GP body with a huge communication power, measured in mega-gigabytes.

Words said, silence kept, drugs given, a demarcation line drawn, an eager-to-please response, a laboratory test not taken – the accumulated stimuli of your 25 million consultations shape Scotland's health concept and form the Scots' illness experience. Doctors can mould health culture by omission, by giving political, commercial and technological forces a free hand – or we can use the 25 million consultations' potential to actively promote a healthy illness culture.

The essential instrument in general practice is 'the word'. The GP is 'the great communicator' of medicine. Spirits and demons are created by words. They are images constructed by thoughts and words. Therefore spirits and demons can only be deconstructed, cured, by words. Once again, we discover the GP's inborn talent for healing the spirits of time.

Angels in the minds of the patients

It is not only demons that sneak into the consulting room with patients, angels fly in with them too. The futurologists forecast that four good spirits will bring general practice in line.[20,21]

The rediscovery of 'I'

The rediscovery of I, as a particular person with a legitimate right to be seen as strange me. The Frank Sinatra refrain 'Do it my way' is the patriotic song of post-modernism. No doctor is more qualified than the GP to meet the patient as an individual – personal doctoring being your very trademark.[22]

The feeling society

Post-modern man is breaking out of the iron cage of rationality. The futurologists predict increasing validity to emotions, sensations, stories, dreams and adventures. The 'blues and soul' of disease – diagnosing and therapy – demand their fair share. Children raised on *Harry Potter* and *The Lord of the Rings* will not thrive in the wasteland of rational biomedicine. The mystery is on, and the GP is medicine's mystery man. Nobody is more competent to combine *scientia cum mysterium* than the GP, whose entity of work has always been the whole human being.

The post-modern *panta rei* scenario

Post-modern mentality is characterised by open-mindedness as opposed to dogmatism. Values of the post-modern culture are uncertainty, many different voices and experiences of reality, and multifaceted descriptions of truth. This could be a description of classic GP mentality. So the post-modern folk-soul will meet a sounding board in the GP's mind.

The enlightened patient

Voltaire switched on the old Enlightenment. The World Wide Web illuminates the new. The enlightened patient needs the GP to make the medical information compatible with their individual life, their particular disease.[23,24] Sir William Osler[25] forecast this general practice value many years ago: 'The man who translates the hieroglyphics of science into the plain language of healing certainly is the most useful.' The patient-centred method demonstrates that we are at the front, prepared to transform the consultation room into a play station for the enlightened patient.[26]

I am not so good with angels. Let me resume my natural attraction to demons.

The demons in the soul of society

We must struggle with the demons in the House of Medicine and in the consulting room. But this is not enough. Our demons do not arise in intracranial isolation. They possess us from outside. Their point of departure is society. Who are the societal demons haunting people's health, producing the clinical challenges in Scotland in 2002? A trinity of political demons prevails in modern Western societies.

The demon of Superman

The prevailing neocapitalist programme demands people to be clones of Superman. We are expected to be productive, creative, flexible, innovative and positive – all the time. The education system as well as modern working life pursue us with Olympic demands: higher, stronger and faster. But neither God, nor Darwin, created us to be as such all the time. The surplus of ambition and the deficiency of time make us sick. Superhuman expectations may be a leading cause for morbidity presented to the GP. So what can we do?

First and foremost, guide the individual patient out of the Superman trap and on to Aristotle's *aurea mediocritas*: the golden middle way of life. Secondly, we should warn society, the politicians, the trade unions and the public against the ravages of the Superman demon.

The demon of Mammon

We dance around the golden calf, but without *joie de vivre*, without health. In our gold rush, we lose life, dignity and freedom. We lose time to read holy books, nature, the eyes of our love, the runes inscribed in our own soul, the mail from our ancestors' spirits. Again we can be tutored by the Basarwa. Possessing worldly goods has always been shunned by the bushmen. The burden of possessions restrains their freedom to move with the animals and the rains, and compromises their very survival. The average personal property of a Basarwa, measured by Harvard researchers, is 12.5 kilograms. The Basarwa have read what we should write on our prescription pads:

> For what shall it profit a man if he shall gain the whole world and lose his own soul?
>
> Mark, 8.36

The demon of Superman and the demon of Mammon nurture a fast-growing child. This is the demon of inequality.

The demon of inequality

Modern Western societies are ridden by the demon of inequality. The differences between people as regards money, dignity, freedom and health are increasing.[27,28]

The Cuban philosopher and freedom fighter, José Marti, said, 'Everything that divides men, everything that specifies, separates or pens them, is a sin against humanity.'[29] And we may add: a threat against human health.

What separates people in Scotland today? Money and pigment cells, economic power and race – as in the Kalahari. It is not only socio-economic status that creates the health divide. The other separating principle in Europe today is race. The most deadly of all ghosts are wandering over Britain and medicine, 'apartheiding' people into superiors and nonentities.[30,31] Too many people in Europe today may recognise that stigma of race. GPs are natural healers of social injustice and racism. The unit of attention in general practice is the individual, never the mass. It is impossible to work as a GP without falling in love with the human element, irrespective of economic power, social prestige, number of melanocytes per mm^2 of skin. The GP discovers 20 times a day that there is more to admire among humans than to despise.

Healing in the House of Scotland

Societal demons take up residence in the minds of doctors, settle in the hearts of patients, and shape and colour clinical images in general practice. General practice should not merely be a passive reflection, a dead echo of modernity. We must feed back to society. The body of GPs must communicate with society, be interactive with the modern health soul.

We are not so clever with that. Traditionally our dedication is framed by the individual patient. We conform to academic norms and perceive mixing with the surrounding world as sinful. We practise medicine in distinguished seclusion from dirty politics, dangerous media and vulgar public debate. Complying with that tradition, we waste our vast potential for political doctoring.

The consulting room represents a unique observation post of society. With their stethoscope, the GP hears the murmurs and sighs of modernity. When the GP has palpated 1000 muscles, they know something about the collective body of their patient population. When the GP has prescribed 1000 boxes of Prozac, they know a lot about the collective soul of the local community.

We work with political affairs transformed to human suffering. The 25 million consultations per year conceal political explosives. But hitherto these have been tacit explosives. We should not let our surgeries be hiding places for society-made sickness. If modern antidepressants were on the market in France in 1789, the Bastille would probably not have been stormed. The GP should learn to read the spurs from medical symptomatology to political aetiology: read them and report them back to society, loud and clear. We must report back the medical inflictions of inequality, unemployment, poverty, racism and superhuman expectations.

Political doctoring

I hope to have brought you from the Kalahari a new dimension of general practice: healing the spirits of time – or political doctoring.

I feel that we, the general practitioners, have an unaccomplished potential, an unfinished job to do when it comes to political doctoring. By political doctoring I do not mean exercising party politics, red or blue, disguised in white. 'Politics' derives from the Greek *polis*, meaning a body of people. So political doctoring is medico-professional activity directed towards the body of people – society. Marshall Marinker recently described the evolution of general practice during the last 50 years:[32]

> The focus of the general practitioner's clinical concern was readjusted, first from diagnosis of disease to the meaning of illness, second, from the illness to the patient, and third, from the patient to the doctor–patient relationship.

Marinker is right, but with a missing link at the end. I would like to add:

> And fourth, from the doctor–patient relationship to the medicine–society interaction.

Our loyalty and priority should always be with the individual patient. But we must not neglect the law of sums:

- Σ Doctors = the culture of medicine
- Σ Patients = the people
- Σ Doctor–patient relationships = medicine–society relationships

The last dance

There is a lot of concern now over the present state of general practice and there are strategic plans for the future. I do not think you need to worry. We have 30 000 years of evidence that no one is more able to survive in the evolution of medicine than general practitioners. You are extreme survivors close to the scorpion and the crocodile – remarkably adaptable and sustainable species. Molecules come and go. Technologies come and go. Even colleges come and go. General practice endures as long as the world goes on. And so do the spirits, the mythology and the demonology of man. To remind you of that eternal truth has been the purpose of my lecture. In the lost world of the Kalahari[33] we can rediscover that spirits are real – that they exist here, now. Colleagues, let us go – boldly go – and dance with the spirits of time.

References

1   Royal College of General Practitioners (1972) *The Future General Practitioner: learning and teaching*. BMJ Books, London.

2   Bleek WHI and Lloyd LC (1911) *Specimens of Bushman Folklore*. Allen, London. [Reprint: Struik, Cape Town, 1968.]

3   Lewis-Williams D and Dowson T (2000) *Images of power: understanding San Rock art*. Struik, Cape Town.

4   Katz R (1982) *Boiling Energy: community healing among Kalahari Kung*. Harvard University Press, Cambridge, MA.

5   Horder J (ed.) (1992) *The Writings of John Hunt*. The Royal College of General Practitioners, London.

6   Heath I (1995) *The Mystery of General Practice*. The Nuffield Provincial Hospitals Trust, London.

7   Howie J (1999) *Patient-centredness and the Politics of Change: a day in the life of academic practice*. The Nuffield Trust, London.

8   McWhinney IR (1996) The importance of being different. *British Journal of General Practice*. **46**: 433–6.

9   Pendleton D (2002) *Values, the College and the General Practitioners*. Lecture given at RCGP 50th Anniversary, London.

10 Burns R (1993) *Selected Poems*. Penguin Books, London.

11 Williams WC (1974) *The Embodiment of Knowledge*. New Directions, New York.

12 Fox T (1965) Purposes of medicine. *Lancet*. **ii**: 801–5.

13 Fanu LF (1999) *The Rise and Fall of Modern Medicine*. Carroll & Graf Publishers, New York.

14 Moynihan R and Smith R (2002) Too much medicine? Almost certainly. *BMJ*. **324**: 859–60.

15 Skrabanek P (1994) *The Death of Humane Medicine and the Rise of Coercive Healthism*. Crowley Esmonde, Suffolk.

16 Hollnagel H and Malterud K (2000) From risk factors to health resources in medical practice. *Medicine and Health Care Philosophy*. **3**: 257–64.

17 Machiavelli N (1952) *The Prince*. William Benton, Chicago.

18 Gaskill H (ed.) (1996) *The Poems of Ossian and Related Works*. Edinburgh University Press, Edinburgh.

19 Beck U (1992) *Risk Society: towards a new modernity*. Sage Publications, London.

20 Mathers N and Rowland S (1997) General practice – a postmodern speciality? *British Journal of General Practice*. **47**: 177–9.

21 Morris DB (1998) *Illness and Culture in the Postmodern Age*. University of California Press, Berkeley.

22 Fugelli P (2001) Trust – in general practice. *British Journal of General Practice.* **51**: 575–9.

23 Ferguson T (2002) From patients to end users. *BMJ.* **324**: 555–6.

24 Hardey M (1999) Doctor in the house – the Internet as a source of lay health information and the challenge to expertise. *Sociology of Health and Illness.* **21**: 820–6.

25 Bean WB (ed.) (1951) *Sir William Osler. Aphorisms from his Bedside Teachings and Writings.* Charles C Thomas Publishers, Springfield.

26 Stewart M, Brown JB, Weston WW *et al.* (1995) *Patient-centred Medicine.* Sage, Newbury Park, CA.

27 Galbraith JK (1992) *The Culture of Contentment.* Houghton Mifflin, Boston, MA.

28 Wilkinson RG (1996) *Unhealthy Societies: the afflictions of inequality.* Routledge, London.

29 Shnookal D and Muniz M (eds) (1999) *José Marti. Reader. Writings on the Americas.* Ocean Press, New York.

30 Commission on the Future of Multi-Ethnic Britain (2000) *The Parekh Report.* Profile Books, London.

31 Coker N (ed.) (2001) *Racism in Medicine: an agenda for change.* King's Fund, London.

32 Marinker M (1998) What is wrong and how do we know it? In: Loudon I, Horder J and Webster C (eds) *General Practice under the National Health Service 1948–1997.* Clarendon Press, Oxford.

33 Post van der L (1962) *The Lost World of the Kalahari.* Penguin, Harmondsworth.

CHAPTER 16

General practice: evolution or revolution?

Claire Jackson and Mayur Lakhani

Introduction

Few people realise the struggle faced by our founders in establishing the Royal College of General Practitioners and getting general practice *accepted* and respected as a discipline. It is often not appreciated how much progress has been made in general practice: a word that is frequently used is 'transformation'. This becomes obvious when one examines the difference now and 50 years ago in how primary healthcare is organised, the quality and standards and range of services provided, the premises from which GPs practise, the use of information management and technology where general practice leads the way in the NHS and the development of research and teaching.

In this chapter we wish to give a selected view of the development of the discipline of general practice and the role that the College played in this. We feel that is important to examine some of the reasons which led to the creation of the College and to explore how this might assist us in coping with the considerable challenges faced by general practice now.

In a sense many of the issues and problems are similar today, although obviously the context and magnitude are different. Members of the health community, particularly outside of academic general practice, may not be familiar with the history, culture and fabric of general practice.

There are many ways to look at the history of general practice over the last 50 years. Modern historical interpretation looks at groups rather than individuals; in this case it was the influence of a number of people who chose to create an institution to further their ideals rather than try to achieve less by individual endeavour. Instead of starting off being part of a larger, existing organisation there was a feeling that what was needed was a revolution: only by forming an entirely new academic body would general practice be able to become a discipline in its own right.

The creation of the College

It could be argued that until the College was founded in 1952 the development of general practice was mainly reactive rather than proactive, with changes being imposed by the State such as the National Insurance Act in 1911 and the creation of the National Health Service in 1948. General practitioners had had no effective influence on these initiatives. After July 1948, GPs were required to provide primary and personal medical care for every citizen registered with them. In addition they became the gateway through which patients normally gained access to specialist hospital care, sickness benefit and many of the other provisions made available under the NHS. The *Lancet*, in an editorial in 1950, wrote:

> General practice is at the crossroads. The general practitioner sees himself being elbowed out of hospital, finds himself more isolated from his colleagues in specialist and consulting practice, is plagued by paper work, and sees little prospect of obtaining those pleasant conditions of work so alluringly offered to him by propagandists for the National Health Service during the years before July 1948.

In the same issue was a report of a survey of practices by Joseph Collings, an Australian academic visiting the country.[1] Although many have argued that the Collings report exaggerated the proportion of negative feeling and poor conditions facing GPs, there is no doubt that there were strong feelings of unhappiness and low morale.

The Collings report was a catalyst for a scientific paradigm shift in thinking. It highlighted the beginnings of the end of what Thomas Kuhn called, in his seminal work on scientific revolutions,[2] 'normal science'; that is, the existing methods and ideology were no longer adequate for the current problems. Collings said, '[There is an] unquestioning acceptance of the traditions of the last century and a failure to think about general practice in contemporary and constructive terms.'[1]

There was an inexorable move towards a 'revolution' by GPs rather than imposed by government or the medical establishment upon the practitioners. In a letter written by John Hunt and Fraser Rose to the *Lancet* and the *BMJ* in 1951,[3] they asked for readers to respond to an idea of creating a College of General Practice:

> It should be able to help practitioners in a great many ways – by supervising their education and postgraduate work, by improving the standard and status of general practice – all at little and no cost to the taxpayer.

Hunt received a great many positive replies. One respondent commented:[4]

> ... it may be asked what could this College do? ... it could be a centre round which general practitioners could rally their standards and ideals. The rehabilitation of general practice is ... a matter for the whole body of general practice to put right within itself. The College could give a lead.

The College was eventually founded in October 1952. *The Practitioner* said, 'The foundation of this College is an outstanding event in the history of British medicine.'[5] There was, however, still an awful lot of work to do to justify this claim. The founders had to create a new discipline for general practice, a new Kuhnian paradigm, '... an entire constellation of beliefs, values, techniques and so on shared by the members of a given community'.[2] It is that which has characterised the last 50 years of general practice and for which the College has played such a leading role.

Not just a club: the meaning of membership

In 1950, a general practice section of the Royal Society of Medicine (RSM) had been formed by some of the same people – such as John Hunt – who were later to be active in founding the College. However, the Council of the RSM had only agreed to the section being founded if it kept strictly to the ideals of the Society:[6] '[The section] would strictly avoid any suspicion that its discussions embraced any matters concerned with the political and ethical as distinct from the technical aspects of general practice.'

Membership of the new College was intended to equate good patient service and maintenance of high standards. Admission to membership depended on fulfilling criteria agreed at the first annual general meeting (November 1953), which included sponsors and evidence about practice. The assessment process was never wholly satisfactory despite attempts to level out inconsistencies. For a while a points system employing differentially weighting criteria was used. Fierce debates ranged within the College during its early years over holding a membership examination. As early as 1954 a questionnaire was sent to all members asking what they thought the criteria for membership should be, and a suggested syllabus and sample examination paper was published in 1955. It was one of a succession of memoranda setting out guidelines for training programmes and how those training others might themselves be taught.

Despite heavy lobbying by George Abercrombie, the membership did not agree to have an exam until 1964. John Horder commented later:[7]

> The examination hurdle prevailed in the end partly because it was believed to guarantee greater knowledge and skill, partly because the rest of the profession (and the public) had to be shown that the College was serious in its intentions for raising quality.

The first examination was held in 1965 with five candidates, all of whom passed. In recent years new routes to membership and Fellowship of the College have been pioneered.

Fellowship by Assessment (FBA) was introduced in 1989. Fellowship of the College was originally awarded to those who had done the institution service or had made an outstanding contribution to medical science in general or general practice in particular. FBA in contrast, as its title suggests, requires the demonstration of defined standards of care. To date, 251 FBAs have been awarded.

Membership by Assessment of Performance (MAP) was introduced in 1999. This is designed to offer a new route to membership for experienced GPs who can show evidence of good quality practice. Candidates have to submit a portfolio of work, containing up to nine submissions, a video assessment or simulated surgery and also have a practice visit by a panel of assessors.

CWC Johnson, writing in the College journal in 1958, has proved remarkably prescient by arguing that:[8]

> If an examination for a diploma is established with high standards, it will inevitably follow that many members must rest content with being members and no more. This itself is a challenge to those of us. More importantly, by cooperating in the accumulation of practice data, the whole body of members could enable any diploma examination to be regarded as an interim one to be replaced in due course by an assessment of the candidate's work in practice over a moderately prolonged period. This would be an epoch-making contribution to the whole of medicine.

Training

The College was very keen to encourage specific training for general practice at all levels. One of the points made by very many of those replying to John Hunt's proposal for a College and who became foundation members was the fact that that they had received little or no training at medical school to prepare them for general practice:[9]

> As a young practitioner still meeting untaught problems peculiar to general practice and attempting to modify a hospital-based medicine to the demands of general practice, I feel that the need of such a college is immense and long overdue.

It was felt important that general practice could and should be taught by general practitioners themselves. As there were no Chairs of General Practice, the faculty structure of the College came into its own. Faculties established links with local medical schools; GPs volunteered to have students spending time in their practices. The Undergraduate Education Committee, under the chairmanship of Richard Scott, published a booklet *On Undergraduate Education and the General Practitioner* in 1958, recommending that a department of education be set up in each medical school. Richard Scott was himself the first holder of a Chair of General Practice, in 1963, at the University of Edinburgh. It was the work of pioneers such as Scott which highlighted the importance of patient- rather than disease-centred care. It is only recently that clinical practice has accepted this methodology long after it was a central tenet of general practice. There are now departments of general practice in all medical schools in Great Britain. In 1974, the Association of University Teachers of General Practice was formed.[10]

The Doctors' Charter in 1966 brought more money into general practice and enabled GPs to employ auxiliary staff, which not only eased the work load but also encouraged the creation of practice teams. The College then set its sights on promoting vocational postgraduate training.

A separate discipline needed separate training, something more than the trainee scheme set up by the Government and BMA in 1952 after the Goodenough Report,[11] enabling newly registered doctors to work for a year in a practice learning about practice organisation and finance. The College wanted special vocational training for general practice within the NHS and ongoing provision for postgraduate study. The need for ongoing training is essential, especially when one considers how the amazing advances in drugs, equipment, diagnostics and surgery over the last 50 years have transformed the way medicine is practised. As early as 1955, the College of General Practice of Canada reported that 90% of prescriptions written by GPs could not have been written 20 years before as the drugs did not exist.

The College set up a Vocational Training Committee and published the definitive *Special Vocational Training for General Practice* in 1965. What gave its guidance particular weight was that its proposals had been piloted within the practices of those preparing the document. The College was well prepared when asked to give evidence to the Royal Commission on Medical Education 1965–8, known as the Todd Report.[12] Thirteen years after the creation of a College of General Practice, they were able to show why general practice was a subject in its own right and put the case for departments of general practice, for VT and for continuing education. The emergence of general practice as a distinct discipline was still not without its critics as the intense growth in medical knowledge had led to a growth in specialities in medicine. The number of specialist sections at the RSM was expanding steadily at this time. Sir Arthur Thompson gave a lecture in 1963 entitled 'Is General Practice Outmoded?'[13] A similar debate exists now with the plans to create GPs with special interests, in which there is a recognised tension with generalism.

The College's case, however, was supported by the Todd Report:[14]

> In recent years much thought has been given by the Royal College of General Practitioners ... and others to the idea of a much more comprehensive scheme of professional training for general practice and we have been impressed by the scheme for ... professional training put to us by the Royal College.

Vocational training was implemented in 1967. Sir Donald Irvine has written about the sense of excitement during the early years of VT and the Vocational Training Subcommittee:[15]

> Its job was to help find solutions to problems as they arose in the experimental schemes and, in general, to act as a fast communication system and forum for ideas for all those most intimately involved.

As another aspect of the discipline of general practice grew up and developed, this *ad hoc* approach was honed and guidelines for scheme organisers, regional advisors and trainers were developed in 1972 in *The Future General Practitioner: learning and teaching*.[16] This controversially tried to predict a job description for a future GP from which educational aims were derived. The definition and aims, slightly amended, were presented by the Leeuwenhorst Group[17] in 1974 to all important bodies concerned with VT in Europe, and were adopted as the basis for GP vocational training across what was then known as the European Economic Community (EEC). By 1973, the responsibility for the selection of vocational trainers moved into the hands of the universities with the newly appointed regional advisors in general practice, who were supported by GP course organisers who ran local training schemes.[18]

It was not until 1974 that the LMC conference agreed that VT should normally be mandatory for those wishing to be principals in the NHS. The necessary regulatory body – the Joint Committee on Postgraduate Training for General Practice – was devised by Ekke Kuenssberg, allegedly while travelling on a London bus. This body has two parent organisations: the College and the General Medical Services Committee of the BMA – now the General Practitioners Committee. The requisite parliamentary legislation was enacted in November 1976 and was implemented in 1981. Training programmes and their supervision, though not now primarily a College remit, continue to be refined and new regulations came into force in 1998.

Quality initiatives

By the 1980s, general practice and the College had achieved many of its goals. David Morrell described this period as some of the happiest years for GPs this century:[19]

> They understood their role, and research and education had helped to solve many of the clinical and organisational problems presented to them. Many practised from purpose-built premises with teams of other primary care professionals.

The College started to turn its attention to the promotion of quality. A quality initiative was published in 1983 which encouraged doctors to define the services they felt their practices should be providing and to monitor their ability to do so. This was followed by *What Sort of Doctor?* in 1985.[20] This tried to analyse what could be assessed as good practice. John Horder characterised *What Sort of Doctor?* as 'courageous' and 'a fundamental landmark because it considers performance the final product rather than knowledge, and because it starts from some agreed commitments about what quality means in medical care'.[7]

The changing nature of general practice

Many will feel a sense of *déjà vu* reading this chapter so far: a sense of not being valued, a state of unhappiness amongst GPs, problems with infrastructure and support in primary healthcare, relentless reform of the health service and the status and standing of general practice. To some extent the struggle continues, and although enormous strides have been made in general practice there is much still to be done. With the changing nature of general practice also come more fundamental questions, based on modern and consumerist values, about the role of medical Royal Colleges and the relationships between the State, the professions and patients. The current climate demands much greater account-ability from doctors. Major areas such as postgraduate medical education, for long the province of medical Royal Colleges, are now subject to major reform by the NHS.

Reversing the decline of professional influence

Throughout this book, a recurring theme has been the importance of organised general practice opinion and professional leadership in shaping developments, e.g. the role the RCGP played in establishing vocational training. We have turned full circle in a sense, with the State and not medical Royal Colleges lead-ing the way in reforming medical practice. This brings home a key issue for professional organisations: the relative decline of their influence. In recent years a shift in power from the profession to the NHS can be discerned in the UK. This process has been a direct challenge to past concepts of professionalism.

Yet, the experience of European primary care has shown that those countries with relatively advanced professional standing for GPs appear to have made most progress: a vitalised and energised profession is important in order to make progress. Health service policy in the UK over the last two decades can be interpreted as replacing internal professional vitality as a driver for progress with external managed direction.

Revitalisation

With such a challenging political climate, it has never been more important than now to have organised general practice opinion. We need to look at how we move general practice forwards. Whilst primary care structures are chang-ing worldwide, general practice should be firmly based on its core principles. It is important to maintain the essence of general practice. An outstanding example of professional endeavour is the document *Good Medical Practice for GPs*,[21] led and produced by the RCGP in conjunction with other general practice organisations. This document laid out for the first time explicit standards for the profession of general practice in the UK. With an ageing population, where co-morbidity is the rule rather than the exception, the unique function of a GP will become even more important. General practice organisations will have a key role in ensuring that a renewal takes place so that GPs continue to become the most influential and important doctors in the NHS.

Conclusion

There will be many people reading this who will, with justification, claim that it is a very partial view of the 50 years of general practice. However, we hope that we have been able to give a glimpse of what it was like 50 years ago and the conditions which led to the creation of the College. The revolutionaries of 50 years ago have created that paradigm: 'an entire constellation of beliefs, values, techniques and so on shared by the members of a given community'.[2] It is a measure of the extent of their success that it is impossible to encompass all of its facets here.

References

1 Collings JS (1950) General practice in England today: reconnaissance. *Lancet.* **i**: 555–85.

2 Kuhn T (1962) *The Structure of Scientific Revolutions.* University of Chicago Press, Chicago.

3 Hunt J and Fraser R (1951) Letter. *Lancet.* **i**: 683.

4 Thwaites J (1952) Letter to BMJ, 27 October 1952.

5 *The Practitioner* (1953) Editorial, January 1953.

6 Council minutes, 20 June 1950. RSM archives.

7 Horder J (1986) Five key events in the history of the RCGP. *London Medicine.* **1**: (3).

8 Johnson CWC (1958) Personal points of view – examinations and the College. *Journal of the Royal College of General Practitioners.* **1** (3): 295.

9 Jones Morgan C (1952) Letter to John Hunt, 17 July 1952. Hunt Archives.

10 This became the Association of University Departments of General Practice and in 2001 the Society for Academic Primary Care.

11 Goodenough Committee (1944) *Report of the Interdepartmental Committee of Medical Schools, Ministry of Health and Department of Health for Scotland.* London.

12 Todd Report (1968) *Royal Commission on Medical Education 1965–68.* HMSO, London.

13 Sir Arthur Thompson (1963) *Is General Practice Outmoded?* Royal Society of Health, 70th Congress, Eastbourne.

14 Ibid. 118, p. 60.

15 Irvine D (1983) Postgraduate education and vocation training Part II 1965–1977. In: Fry J, Hunt JH and Pinsent RJFH (eds) *A History of the Royal College of General Practitioners: the first twenty-five years,* p. 98. MTP, Lancaster.

16 Royal College of General Practitioners (1972) *The Future General Practitioner: learning and teaching.* BMJ Books, London. [Later republished RCGP.]

17 The Leeuwenhorst Group became the New Leeuwenhorst Group in 1982 and in 1992 the European Academy of Teachers in General Practice (EURACT).

18 Periera Gray D (1998) Postgraduate training. In: Webster C, Horder J and Loudon I (eds) *General Practice Under the National Health Service 1948–1997,* p. 191. Oxford University Press, Oxford.

19 Morrell D (1998) Introduction and overview. In: Webster C, Horder J and Loudon I (eds) *General Practice Under the National Health Service 1948–1997,* p. 13. Oxford University Press, Oxford.

20 Royal College of General Practitioners (1985) *What Sort of Doctor?* Reports from General Practice No. 23. RCGP, London.

21 Royal College of General Practitioners and the General Practitioners Committee (2002) *Good Medical Practice for GPs.* RCGP, London.

Index